DUMBBELL TRAINING FOR STRENGTH AND FITNESS

D0206771

Matt Brzycki and Fred Fornicola

Blue River Press
Indianapolis

LCCN: 2006920694

Cover designed by Mark Collins

Printed in the United States of America
10 9 8 7 6 5 4 3

Published in the United States by
BLUE RIVER PRESS
2222 Hillside Avenue, Suite 100
Indianapolis, Indiana 47218, USA
www.cardinalpub.com

DEDICATIONS

Matt Brzycki: *To my lovely wife, Alicia, and our adorable son, Ryan. Thanks for being there.*

Fred Fornicola: *To my wife and best friend, Lori, who has always supported me in everything that I do and my daughter, Alexa, who gives me the greatest gift I could ever have every time she calls me "Daddy."*

ACKNOWLEDGMENTS

The authors extend a sincere thanks to these individuals, without whom the book wouldn't have been possible:

Mark Collins of Bright Ideas Graphics for designing the front and back covers.

Holly Kondras for doing the layout and design of the book and coordinating the project with the printer.

Steve Baldwin, Drew Baye, Randy Berning, Michael Bradley, Jim Bryan, Luke Carlson, Brian Conatser, Michael De Joseph, Jeff Friday, Jason Hadeed, Chip Harrison, Aaron Hillman, Gregg Humphreys, Sunir Jossan, Tom Kelso, Paul Kennedy, Sam Knopik, Aaron Komarek, Kristopher Kotch, Mike Lawrence, Ken Leistner, Ken Mannie, John Mikula, Willis Paine, Adam Rankin, Jeff Roudebush, Doug Scott, Mike Shibinski, Rob Spector and Scott Swanson for contributing most of the workouts that are found throughout the book.

Raymundo Abayon, Tony Alexander, Allison Bibbo, Steve Bibbo, Charity Bonfiglio, James Dong, Alexa Fornicola, Lori Fornicola, Lauren Green, Paul Harker, Dee Haege, Tom Haege, Darryl Hughes, Rhonda Johnson, Tom Kelso, Mark Lewin, Andrew Markoff, Joseph Mislan, Michael New, David Rivera, Sharon Rodgers, Doug Scott, Todd Simmons, Bob Vale, Janice Vale, Dawne Weber and Kevin Weber for volunteering their time to pose for the photographs that appear in the book.

Tom Kelso for providing a photograph that appears in Chapter 9.

Michigan State University Spartan Football for providing two photographs, one that appears in Chapter 1 and the other in Chapter 10.

Cybex International, Incorporated, for providing the artwork that appears in Chapters 3 - 8 and Appendices A and B.

Except as noted previously, all photographs were taken or provided by Matt Brzycki and Fred Fornicola.

TABLE OF CONTENTS

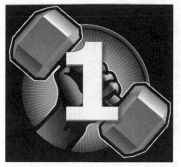 # WHY DUMBBELL TRAINING?

Believe it or not, there was a time when the fitness world wasn't dominated by high-tech equipment as it is today. Years ago, the barbell was the equipment of choice for most strength and fitness enthusiasts – much as it is today. But even before the barbell came the dumbbell, a distinct device of early exercise that held a lofty place as one of the original pieces of equipment for developing might and muscle.

The fact of the matter is that people have been using dumbbells – or dumbbell-like objects – since ancient times to improve their strength and fitness. Way back in the fifth century B.C., Greek athletes employed halteres or "jumping weights." The oblong-shaped halteres were made of stone or lead and used by jumpers in competition. Prior to the takeoff, they were held as if grasping the handle of a shield and positioned behind the athletes. At the takeoff, the athletes extended the halteres forward in order to propel them further. At the time, ancient athletes also developed their strength for competitions by training with the halteres. While holding the weights, they did exercises that resembled the bicep curl, lunge and some type of back extension. The halteres were a valuable mainstay as a training tool that would be modified and improved over the centuries.

The importance of using exercise to increase strength and fitness became a necessity in many cultures – and not just for men. A mosaic that dates back to the second century clearly shows a bikini-clad woman doing some type of physical activity with a pair of hand-held weights.

It wasn't until the middle of the 18th century in merry olde England that the name "dumbbell" was given to the object with two "bells." The bells were made by taking church-like bells and removing their clappers. They then were secured to both ends of a short handle. During this period, anyone who couldn't speak was referred to as "dumb." Some researchers think that because the bell made no sound, it was christened a "dumb bell."

Here's another historical nugget: Benjamin Franklin is renowned for his keen mind but he also took care of his body. In a letter to his son in August 1772, Franklin explained how he preferred "strenuous exercise" that was done "in short periods of time" – which, by the way, sure sounds a lot like an endorsement of High-Intensity Training (HIT)! He noted that the value of exercise could be judged by the "amount of warmth it produced in the body" and that dumbbell training was "an excellent way to produce bodily warmth." Clearly, Ben Franklin was no dumbbell.

At any rate, the early dumbbells were rather unsuitable as a standard piece of equipment. It was difficult to find bells that were different sizes and weights. This made them cost prohibitive. Eventually, the shot-loaded dumbbell was created by taking two hollow steel balls and securing one to each end of a short handle. Each ball had a plug that could be unscrewed to add or remove steel shot and voilá, the first adjustable dumbbell was born! This advancement ultimately led to the modern-day dumbbell with which we're more familiar. While on the subject, dumbbells now come in several different types including round and hex.

No doubt, the dumbbell had made its mark in fitness as being a highly effective, convenient and suitable piece of equipment for most anyone to use – even for one of our founding fathers!

ADVANTAGES AND DISADVANTAGES

All exercise equipment has its share of good points and bad points. And as a training tool, the dumbbell is no exception. Let's take a glimpse at the advantages and disadvantages of dumbbells. Since the dumbbell is most closely related to the barbell, many of the discussions will make comparisons between the two modalities.

Advantages of Dumbbells

There are many important advantages of using dumbbells. Here are some things to consider:

Independent Workload

A major advantage of using dumbbells is that it forces each of your limbs to work independently of the other. Most individuals are stronger (and more flexible) on one side of their body than the other side. Usually, this isn't a significant difference. But when there's a gross difference in the strength between limbs, the use of dumbbells is highly recommended. This is also an important consideration for rehabilitative strength training. In this case, an individual may even have to work one limb at a time while using a lighter weight for the weaker limb.

Relative Safety

Another big plus of dumbbells is that they allow you to train alone in a reasonably safe manner. Here's a perfect example: When performing a supine (flat bench) press with a barbell, you should get a "spot" from a competent spotter or training partner or use a safety rack. Doing so will

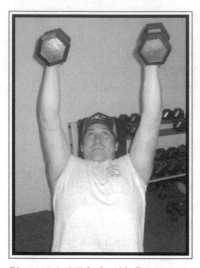

Figure 1.1: With dumbbells, you can train confidently and safely to muscular fatigue without the need of a spotter.

reduce the potential for an unexpected mishap such as losing your grip or being trapped under the weighted bar. This is a very dangerous situation and one that shouldn't be taken lightly; it literally could be life threatening. Researchers looked at data on patients who were admitted to the emergency rooms of hospitals from 1978-98. In that 20-year period, 34 deaths were attributed to weight training and 22 (67%) of the lifters were alone at the time of injury. In one of those fatalities, the lifter died from asphyxiation after the barbell fell onto his neck. The take-home message: Don't become a statistic.

With dumbbells, you cannot get "stuck" since you can simply lower the weights to the floor thereby avoiding the possibility of serious injury. And speaking of the supine press – or any of its variants for that matter such as the incline press and decline press – doing the exercise to muscular fatigue with a barbell requires the presence of a competent spotter. But with dumbbells, you can train confidently and safely to muscular fatigue without that requirement.

Added Variety

Yet another advantage of using dumbbells is that they can provide variety to your workouts. Remember, every exercise that can be performed with a barbell can also be performed with dumbbells. For the most part, dumbbells can be incorporated into your workouts as easily as barbells and, in certain cases, make for a better alternative.

For example, you can do the bent-over row with a barbell using both arms at the same time but this puts your lower back in a precarious position. It's much better to do the bent-over row with one arm at a time using the non-exercising arm for support to stabilize your torso and, thus, your lower back.

Also keep in mind that there are quite a few exercises that you can do with dumbbells but not with a barbell. This includes the lateral raise, bent-over raise, internal rotation, external rotation, dorsi flexion and side bend. Several other exercises can be performed with a barbell but they're less awkward to do with dumbbells. For instance, it's much more cumbersome to do the pullover and front raise with a barbell.

Performance Versatility

Related to additional variety is the fact that dumbbells also allow you to utilize multiple performance variations that are literally impossible to do with a barbell. The conventional approach is to do repetitions with two limbs at the same time (bilateral training); with dumbbells, you can also do repetitions with one limb at a time (unilateral training). Using the overhead press as an example, you can perform a set with your left arm first followed by a set with your right arm.

In addition to having the option of using one limb at a time, you can also do your repetitions in an alternating fashion. Let's look at three different ways to do the ever-popular bicep curl with dumbbells in an alternating fashion:

1. Perform one repetition (raising and lowering the dumbbell) with your right arm and then one repetition (raising and lowering the dumbbell) with your left arm. Repeat this pattern until you complete the set.

2. Raise both dumbbells to the mid-range position (your arms bent). Perform one repetition (lowering and raising the dumbbell) with your right arm and then one rep-

etition (lowering and raising the dumbbell) with your left arm. Repeat this pattern until you complete the set.

3. Raise the dumbbell to the mid-range position with your right arm. Lower the dumbbell to the start/finish position with your right arm while simultaneously raising the dumbbell to the mid-range position with your left arm. Raise the dumbbell back to the mid-range position with your right arm while simultaneously lowering the dumbbell to the start/finish position with your left arm. Repeat this pattern until you complete the set. (With this style, you must focus on performing the repetitions without swinging your body and/or using an excessive amount of momentum.)

At first glance, it may appear as if the first and second examples are the same. Well, they're similar but the subtle difference is actually significant. In the first example, one arm does a complete repetition while the other arm stays in the start/finish position, essentially performing no work other than to simply maintain a grip on the dumbbell; in the second example, one arm does a complete repetition while the other arm stays in the mid-range position, essentially performing an isometric or a static contraction. Needless to say, this latter action makes for a much more intense exercise.

In discussing the various methods of multiple-performance styles, it's important to consider the versatility that an adjustable bench can add to dumbbell training.

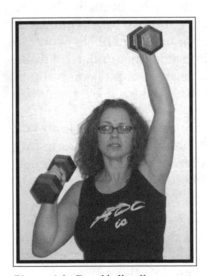

Figure 1.2: Dumbbells allow you to utilize multiple performance variations that are literally impossible to do with a barbell.

Depending on the number of adjustment levels of the bench, the variety of angles affords an enormous amount of diversity. Here's a perfect illustration: Dan Riley, the Strength and Conditioning Coach of the Houston Texans, has popularized an innovative sequence of exercises for the chest, shoulders and triceps that he refers to as the "dumbbell elevator." Essentially, the dumbbell elevator involves doing one set of each exercise to muscular fatigue at each level (or "floor") of an adjustable bench. The number of levels depends on the bench. (One 0-90 adjustable bench can be positioned at six different levels: at 0, 18, 36, 54, 72 and 90 degrees.) You can start at the bottom floor and take the elevator to the top floor, stopping at each level to do a set. Or, you can start at the top floor and do it the other way around. If you face the bench, you can do a few levels for pulling/rowing movements as well.

Greater Contractions

With dumbbells, you can produce a greater contraction of the targeted muscles in certain exercises. This makes the exercise more productive.

Here's an example: The main function of the chest muscles – or in weight-room lingo, the "pecs" – is to pull the arms across the body. When you do a pressing (or pushing) movement with dumbbells for your chest – the supine press, incline press or decline press – you can gradually bring your hands closer together as you raise the weight. This action produces a greater contraction of your chest muscles, meaning that more muscle fibers are engaged which can lead to increased strength and muscular development. Obviously, you cannot bring your hands closer together as you raise a barbell.

Here's another example: One of the main functions of the trapezius is shoulder elevation (shrugging the shoulders as if to say, "I don't know.") An excellent exercise for isolating this muscle is the shrug. When this exercise is done with a barbell, the weight must be positioned in front of your shoulders. This restricts the contraction of your trapezius. When this exercise is done with dumbbells, the weight can be positioned at your sides. This allows you to obtain a greater contraction of your trapezius.

Weight Distribution

Another consideration that comes into play with a few exercises is the weight distribution. Two exercises in which this is a factor are the shrug and deadlift. In both of these exercises, the barbell must be positioned in front of your shoulders. This causes your shoulders to be pulled forward (not to mention the fact that the bar rides up and down your upper legs as you do the exercises). Performing the exercises with dumbbells held at your sides distributes the weight in a manner that reduces the stress in your front shoulders and lower back.

Hand/Grip Positions

Dumbbells give you the unrestricted freedom to change the position of your hands to best suit your natural mechanics and comfort level. So you can do a bicep curl with dumbbells using a traditional grip (with your palms facing up), a "parallel grip" (with your palms facing each other), a reverse grip (with your palms facing down) or even a grip that's somewhere in between.

This may be an important consideration for some people, especially those who experience joint pain during certain exercises. Many times, there's less orthopedic stress when you opt for a different hand position. Suppose that you have slight pain or discomfort in your shoulder when doing the supine press with a barbell. Perhaps this is due to a lack of flexibility in your shoulder joint or maybe your shoulder is or was injured. In any case, it's quite possible that simply changing the position of your hands from that used with a barbell to a parallel grip with dumbbells will allow you to perform the exercise in a relatively pain-free manner.

Here's why: When the position of your hands is changed so that they face each other, it causes the head of your humerus (your upper-arm bone) to rotate laterally which may reduce the stress on your shoulder joint. Besides the supine press, other exercises in which this tactic can offer orthopedic relief for the shoulder joint include the incline press, decline press, bent-over row, bench row, overhead press, shrug and deadlift.

Space Requirements

If you train at home, a big advantage of dumbbells is that they take up very little space. This is especially true of high-tech, self-contained systems such as the PowerBlock®, Stamina Versa Bell™ and Bowflex® SelectTech™ Dumbbells. Consider this: One "set" of the PowerBlock® can be adjusted from 5 - 45 pounds in five-pound increments. In effect, then, it has nine pairs of dumbbells that would provide a combined weight of 450 pounds. Yet, the set only takes up three square feet of space.

Improved Efficiency

Another important advantage of dumbbells is that you can train in a highly efficient manner. As you'll see in subsequent chapters, structuring workouts that are based solely on dumbbells is very easy. When training with a high level of intensity (or effort), you can complete your workout in about 30 minutes or less. Workouts are even more efficient with selectorized dumbbells: Adjustments in the weight literally take seconds.

Greater Affordability

Perhaps the best feature of all – at least for those who train in the comfort of their homes – is that dumbbells are quite affordable. The price of dumbbells can range anywhere from $0.30 per pound for used ones to about $1.50 per pound for new, depending on the style and brand. So for the most part, outfitting a home gym with a nice set of dumbbells can be done for a few hundred dollars. (For more information on training in your home, refer to *The Essential Guide to At-Home Training.*)

Disadvantages of Dumbbells

As noted earlier, all equipment has at least some disadvantages. The good news is that they can be countered effectively. Let's look at the disadvantages of dumbbells and see how you can overcome them.

Progression Increments

One drawback of dumbbells is that most of them come in five-pound increments. Lighter dumbbells are available in 2.5-pound increments or smaller but aren't always available in commercial gyms. Because of the five-pound increments, progressing to the next level of weight is sometimes impractical. For instance, suppose that your repetition goal in the bicep curl is 12 and today you did 12 repetitions with 25 pounds. Since you reached your repetition goal, you should increase the resistance for your next workout. But the next pair of dumbbells "in line" is the 30-pounders. A five-pound increase in resistance doesn't seem too significant. But you should think of progressions in relative terms, not absolute terms. Here, a five-pound increase from 25 pounds to 30 pounds is actually a 20% increase in resistance which is quite significant. Your muscles and joints might not be prepared for such a sizeable jump in resistance. Furthermore, increasing the resistance too much may cause your technique to suffer. And when using a heavier weight, any small flaws in your technique can be greatly magnified.

So, it's important to be able to micro-load in smaller increments. As the name implies, a micro-load is a small amount of resistance that allows you to progress in a more reasonable and manageable fashion. Fortunately, there are a few ways to micro-load dumbbells. One way is to wear ankle weight on your wrists. Using 25-pound dumbbells while wearing 1.25-pound weights on your wrists makes for 26.25 pounds of resistance – which represents a 5% increase in resistance. This micro-loading protocol can be used until you progress to the 30-pound dumbbells.

Another way to make more manageable increases in resistance is to use a PlateMate®. These are small weights with magnets embedded in them. The magnetized weights can be secured to the sides of a dumbbell. They come in two shapes for dumbbells – hex and "donut" – and weigh as little as 5/8 pound.

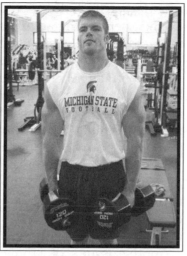

Figure 1.3: Always have a solid foundation and set your body in a "strong" position before picking up or putting down dumbbells.

Positioning Dumbbells

Because dumbbells can be cumbersome – especially the heavy ones – you must use great care in getting them into position prior to performing the actual exercise. Remember, strength training is done to improve your strength and fitness and make your muscles less susceptible to injury. As such, you don't want to get hurt in the process. So take special care in planning and practice how to handle dumbbells properly and safely, especially those of heavier weight.

When using dumbbells, make sure that your body is always in good alignment. This means that you don't twist or reach too far to pick up or put down dumbbells. Always, always, always have a solid foundation. Start by positioning your feet shoulder-width apart. Stay flexed and tight through your hips, legs, mid-section and, finally, your torso. Set your body in a "strong" position before picking up or putting down dumbbells and take extra care not to round your back; this could injure your lower back.

When performing an exercise such as a supine press or an incline press, make sure to follow the previous instructions prior to sitting on the bench. Make sure that you're securely situated on the bench and rest the dumbbells on your upper legs just above your knees. To get into the start/finish position, use your legs to assist your arms by gently raising your legs while simultaneously pulling the weight toward you with your arms. You can do this with one dumbbell at a time (which works well for the incline press and overhead press) or both dumbbells at once (which works well for the supine press and decline press). Sit back carefully and perform the exercise. After completing the exercise, place the dumbbells back on your legs and stand up.

Another issue – one that few of us would mind having – is that heavier dumbbells are longer and bulkier than lighter dumbbells and, as a result, more difficult to use. This depends on the exercise and individual, of course. Regardless, the fact is that a larger-sized dumbbell – larger in weight and/or length – is harder to control than a smaller-sized dumbbell. In addition, a heavier dumbbell makes it more difficult to perform the exercise correctly with a desirable range of motion. This can create an unsafe environment that's conducive to injury. It's recommended to err on the side of caution and find an alternative exercise or take another approach. Some effective tactics are to use a slower speed of movement, incorporate pre-exhaustion techniques or perform higher repetitions (all of which will be discussed in Chapter 9). These tactics will limit the amount of weight that's needed for a particular exercise without sacrificing results.

Incorrect Resistance

History is unclear as to whether or not Isaac Newton was as fond of dumbbell training as Ben Franklin. But Newton did teach us a thing or two about gravity. For starters, gravity is a force that pulls straight down. Because of the effects of gravity, exercises in which dumbbells move in a vertical plane (straight up and down) – such as the overhead press, bent-over row, shrug and calf raise – can be highly effective. With you pushing or pulling the dumbbells straight up and gravity acting straight down, the application of the resistance is absolutely perfect.

The problem is that not all exercises with dumbbells are linear; many are rotary. When rotary exercises are done with dumbbells, the resistance can feel very light in some positions and very heavy in others. A perfect example is the lateral raise. The easiest part of the exercise – where you have the most leverage – is when your arms are perpendicular to the floor; the hardest part of the exercise – where you have the least leverage – is when your arms are parallel to the floor. As you raise your arms, you lose leverage. When you do the lateral raise with dumbbells, you must use a resistance that you can handle in your weakest position – where your arms are parallel to the floor. Think about it: If you use a resistance that you can handle in your strongest position – where your arms are perpendicular to the floor – you wouldn't be able to raise the dumbbells away from your sides. So the resistance is only correct when your arms are parallel to the floor. In all other positions along the range of motion, the resistance is incorrect; it's too light.

Despite this inherent drawback, most rotary exercises can be effective. However, several rotary exercises cannot be done in a meaningful and comfortable way with dumbbells. To do the leg curl and leg extension with dumbbells, for example, you'd have to strap the weights to your feet. Besides being terribly awkward, the resistance would feel either too heavy or too light as you perform the exercise. But here's the good news: The primary muscles that are used in the leg curl and leg extension – the hamstrings and quadriceps, respectively – are used in most multiple-joint exercises for your hips. The hip adduction is another rotary exercise that cannot be performed with dumbbells in a meaningful and comfortable way. However, the muscles that are used in that exercise – the hip adductors or "inner thigh" – are used as stabilizers in most multiple-joint exercises for your hips. This is quite fortunate since these muscles – particularly the hamstrings and inner thigh – are highly prone to injury and strengthening them goes a long way in safeguarding them.

But the most important muscles – at least as it pertains to catastrophic injury – are those that surround your cervical spine or neck. Therefore, those who are involved in any type of contact sport - such as football, rugby, judo and wrestling - are advised to perform strengthening exercises for their necks. Even if you don't participate in a contact sport, having a stronger neck can offer substantial protection against a stiff neck, a neck sprain/strain (a "whiplash") or an injury that's much more severe such as damage to the spinal column. Two popular exercises for strengthening the neck are neck flexion and neck extension. Unfortunately, these are rotary exercises that cannot be performed with dumbbells in a meaningful and comfortable way. The posterior (back) part of your neck is involved somewhat during the shrug. But the anterior (front) part of your neck cannot be exercised with dumbbells in a meaningful and comfortable way. As a result, you're encouraged to find an appropriate means of training your neck - via a machine or manual resistance – especially if you participate in activities that make your neck susceptible to injury.

The moral of the story is that you can overcome the limitations of certain exercises by employing a well-rounded program. Such a program would include a variety of exercises that target the muscles from different angles.

Grip Fatigue

A drawback of training with dumbbells – and barbells, for that matter – is that it can take a heavy toll on your grip. Understand that there's nothing wrong with getting "extra" work for your gripping muscles. But grip fatigue could be a limiting factor in your workout.

Obviously, you can minimize grip fatigue by simply strengthening the muscles that affect your forearms, wrists, hands and fingers. Something else that's often recommended to avoid grip fatigue is to use wrist straps. While it doesn't sound like a big deal, using wrist straps is a serious point of contention. Some fitness authorities and enthusiasts are adamantly opposed to their use because they think that wrist straps provide artificial assistance in holding onto the weight.

Is this a legitimate concern? While wrist straps do offer "artificial assistance," their use is justified if you have difficulty in maintaining your grip on the dumbbells. Here's an example: Suppose that you have to stop after doing 10 repetitions in the shrug when you begin to lose your grip. In this case, you cannot adequately work your trapezius because your gripping muscles are a limiting factor. Or look at it this way: Without wrist straps, you "underwork" your trapezius.

Besides the shrug, the use of wrist straps may be warranted in the deadlift, bench row, bent-over row and upright row. But to reiterate, wrist straps shouldn't be used in lieu of doing exercises to strengthen your gripping muscles.

Range of Motion

Some dumbbell exercises may not provide direct resistance over a full range of motion. For instance, the main muscle of the upper back – the latissimus dorsi or more simply, the "lats" – is capable of moving your upper arm through a range of motion of as much as 270 degrees. With a dumbbell pullover, direct resistance for the lats is only provided through about 100 degrees. This means that not all of the muscle fibers of the lats are engaged.

This isn't a drawback, however, when a well-rounded program is implemented. For example, although the pullover with a dumbbell provides direct resistance over a limited range of motion, including another exercise in your program for your lats – such as a bent-over row or bench row – can help you overcome this constraint.

THE BOTTOM LINE

In one form or another, dumbbells have been used for thousands of years. When used properly, safely, intensely and infrequently, dumbbells can be extremely effective and efficient. This type of dumbbell training will be illustrated in the forthcoming chapters of this book.

REFERENCES:

Jones, C. S., C. Christensen and M. Young. 2000. Weight training injury trends: a 20-year survey. *The Physician and Sports Medicine* 28 (7): 61-52, 65-66, 71-72.

Riley, D. 2004. Dumbbell elevator routine. Available at www.houstontexans.com/fitness/news_detail.php?PRKey=1270.

Riley, D. and J. Arapoff. 1998. Don't make fun of a dumbbell . . . it works! *Coach and Athletic Director* 67 (10): 56-58.

Todd, J. 1995. From Milo to Milo: a history of barbells, dumbbells, and Indian clubs. *Iron Game History* 3 (6): 4-16.

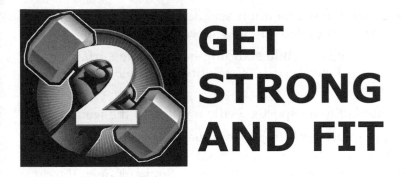

GET STRONG AND FIT

There are many different approaches that you can use to improve your strength and fitness. Your task is to pick the one that's most appropriate for your needs. When deciding on how to best improve your strength and fitness, you must ask yourself these two main questions:

Is the approach safe?

Is the approach effective and efficient?

Taking a closer look at the basis of these two questions will help you to come up with some sensible answers.

SAFETY

The number one concern when training is safety. Your goal should be to improve your strength and fitness, not to jeopardize your orthopedic health. The issue of safety manifests itself in a wide variety of forms. For instance, your approach isn't as safe as possible if you . . .

- include exercises that are ballistic or "explosive" in nature

- perform low-repetition sets (less than about five repetitions) with relatively fast speeds of movement
- do exercises while standing on unstable surfaces (such as a balance board or stability ball) or balance on one limb
- attempt to do sport-specific training in the weight room
- use improper lifting technique

More will be said later about these and other activities but for now, understand that they can yank open the door to injury. Potential injuries include trauma to the lumbar spine (the lower back) and damage to the joints and soft tissues (the muscles, tendons and ligaments) from excessive shearing forces. Incidentally, injuries that occur from exercising in an unsafe manner may not be outwardly or immediately apparent. In other words, injuries might not be realized within the walls of a gym; instead, they may appear at some point down the road. Often, these conditions can occur over time from the cumulative effect of unsafe activities and may materialize when it's least expected such as participating in some type of unrelated physical activity or doing something as simple as bending over to tie your shoes, taking out the garbage or raking leaves.

To reiterate: Many traditional activities – such as doing explosive exercises, low-repetition sets and certain exercises while standing on unstable surfaces – can be cancerous to your body. To paraphrase John Dunn, the

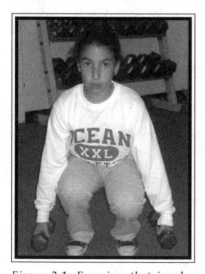

Figure 2.1: Exercises that involve holding onto a resistance (such as dumbbells) should be done on a solid, stable surface.

Strength and Conditioning Coach of the Washington Redskins, "Your body is like a tire. You're only given so much tread and when it wears out, you're all done." Because safety is such a critical concern with your strength training, it's worth examining the aforementioned issues and a few others in greater detail. Along the way, the discussions will expose some myths and misconceptions in strength and fitness that continue to linger. So without further ado, let's see how you can keep the tread on your tire.

Explosive Training

A prevalent belief that has been propagated for decades is that you can increase your power and/or explosiveness by doing certain things in the weight room such as performing "explosive"-type movements, training with relatively low repetitions and lifting a weight as quickly as possible. It's thought that doing these and other types of "explosive training" in the weight room will preferentially engage the so-called "fast-twitch" muscle fibers. Movements that are done with dumbbells in an explosive fashion include the power clean and snatch.

This begs the question, "What is explosiveness?" Well, not what you may think. According to Ken Mannie, the Strength and Conditioning Coach at Michigan State University, "What we refer to as 'explosiveness' is often actually great reaction time."

This stated, there are no exercises, gadgets or gizmos that will make you more explosive. Nor will you need to train in a certain manner to target a specific muscle-fiber type. According to Dr. Michael Wolf, it's the intensity or force requirements that determine which muscle fibers – and how many – are used, not the speed of movement. There's no consistent evidence that proves that the speed of movement dictates the recruitment of muscle fibers. One thing is for sure, though: Lifting weights in a quick fashion will lessen the degree that a muscle is stimulated and also raise the likelihood of injury – both of which are counterproductive to your goals. More will be discussed on that topic in just a bit.

It's also important to realize that performing a movement such as the power clean or snatch with a dumbbell, for example, requires an extremely high level of skill. Even when done with good technique, these exercises can place a tremendous amount of orthopedic stress on your body. You'll reduce your risk of injury by following a program that embeds safe exercises within the protocols and applications that are outlined in this book.

So how do you become more explosive? Well, you need to do two things. First, you must strengthen all of your major muscles. You should do this in a manner that's safe (as well as effective and efficient). Second, you must improve your reaction time by becoming more skilled. You can do this by practicing the intended sport skill for thousands and thousands of task-specific repetitions – until the skill becomes second nature. Dr. Ken Leistner, a strength coach and chiropractor from Long Island (New York), adds that " . . . one needs to train the muscles necessary for his or her particular sport [or activity], make those structures as strong as possible, and then ally this increased strength with the skills of the sport [or activity]."

Low-Repetition Sets

Another safety consideration is the number of repetitions that are performed in a set. Proponents of explosive lifting usually recommend lower repetition ranges (less than about five). Supposedly, this is done to preferentially engage the fast-twitch muscle fibers with the underlying premise that an individual should lift as rapidly as possible with heavier loads. As mentioned previously, the notion that you can selectively recruit certain muscle fibers by using fast speeds of movement is unproven.

Here again, the potential for injury is a major concern. In particular, "maxing out" – attempting to do one repetition with as much weight as possible – is potentially dangerous. When trying to improve strength and fitness, it serves little purpose other than to stroke the ego. "Maxing out" is often done solely to *demonstrate* strength while doing very little to *develop* it.

The simple truth is that there are much safer and more effective ways to demonstrate *and* develop strength simultaneously. Performing 20 repetitions of the deadlift with 100-pound dumbbells is certainly an impressive feat that demonstrates

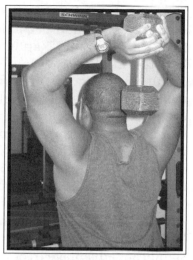

Figure 2.2: *Your muscles should do as much of the work as possible, not momentum.*

strength. But at the same time, this type of effort develops strength (as well as metabolic fitness).

Note: Low-repetition sets can be done in a safe manner provided that the speed of movement is relatively slow. A five-repetition set that takes a handful of seconds to complete is unsafe; a five-repetition set that takes 40 seconds or more to complete is not.

Instability Training

A belief that's erroneous as well as unsafe is that there's a need to perform certain exercises – or better stated, "maneuvers" – on unstable surfaces in order to develop the "core" and become more "functional." Doing exercises for what's currently referred to as the "core" – the abdominals and lower back or, collectively, the mid-section – is nothing new, although some organizations and self-proclaimed "experts" would have you believe that this is a recent breakthrough or that they invented "core training" or "functional training." Indeed, people have been developing their "core" and becoming more "functional" for centuries. Recall from Chapter 1 that the Greeks were using halteres "back in the day," specifically around the fifth century B.C. Among other things, they did various movements with hand-held weights – including a type of back extension – to develop their abdominals and lower back thereby increasing the strength of their "core" and making their entire body more "functional." In fact, if you ever did any type of exercises for your abdominals and lower back, then you did "core training."

Doing an exercise while standing on an unstable surface – or standing on one leg while simultaneously twisting your body with a weighted object in hand – offers absolutely no significant advantage over doing an exercise for your midsection in a traditional manner to develop your "core" or become more "functional." It does, however, increase your risk of injury based on the lack of stability and the undesirable forces that are placed on your joints and soft tissues – not to mention the fact that it does nothing whatsoever to improve strength through a full range of motion. Also of note are countless anecdotal reports of a ball bursting while an individual is performing exercises on it while holding weights or weighted objects.

Remember, these unorthodox and unsafe exercises are merely trendy and sexy approaches that complicate the relatively simple act of becoming stronger, fit and more "functional" throughout your entire body. Developing your "core" is no more than training your abdominals and lower back through a full range of motion with simple yet effective exercises that, for reasons of safety, are done on a solid, stable surface while using proper lifting techniques. As a way to provide variety in your program, you can certainly do some exercises on a stability ball with your bodyweight as the resistance. Understand, however, that these exercises have limitations. In short, trying to build your "core" on an unstable surface makes about as much sense as trying to build your house on quicksand.

Sport-Specific Training

Another fetish that has no valid basis is doing sport-specific training in the weight room. There are emotional claims from the "experts" that simulating sport skills in the weight room will "carry over" to the playing field. (Here, the "playing field" can be taken literally to mean a football field, basketball court, swimming pool and so on or figuratively to mean the performance of simple, everyday tasks.)

To illustrate, it has been recommended that the squat should be done by an offensive lineman to simulate exploding forward to block an opponent and by an outside hitter to simulate exploding upward to block a volleyball. In theory, this seems to have merit but it actually fails miserably in application. For one thing, doesn't it smell just a wee bit fishy that one exercise can simulate two distinctly different sport skills that have two distinctly different movement patterns? And this is just the tip of the proverbial iceberg: The squat is supposedly "specific" to dozens of other sport skills with vastly different movement patterns.

The squat is a great exercise for strengthening your hips and legs, provided that you're biomechanically suited to do the exercise in a safe fashion. (Having relatively short legs and a short spine make the exercise safer.) However, the squat doesn't duplicate, simulate, mimic or resemble anything other than a squat. Dr. Leistner adds, "The worth of an exercise is determined by its ability to strengthen a muscular structure for the sport [activity] in question, not by its resemblance to actual on the field maneuvers."

As noted earlier, it's important to strengthen all of your major muscles and practice the intended sport skill. Whether a person becomes stronger in the lower body by performing a squat, deadlift, lunge or leg press really doesn't matter. What does matter is that the muscles that are needed to perform a given skill are being strengthened.

Sport-specific training also attempts to simulate sport skills through the use of weighted objects such as a dumbbell, medicine ball, weighted vest or other heavier-than-normal implements. Take, for example, a quarterback who wants to increase the strength of his shoulder with the intent that this will improve the velocity of his throws. To do this, he decides to simulate his throwing motion with a five-pound dumbbell. Although the intent is well meaning, here's what will happen: The heavier and unfamiliar weight of the dumbbell will cause him to learn different mechanics. Essentially, his neuromuscular system – his nerves and muscles – will learn a similar but new skill: throwing a five-pound dumbbell. When he returns to throwing a regulation football – which is obviously a much different size, shape and weight than a five-pound dumbbell – he'll find that his mechanics are off and he must relearn how to throw a regulation football. But the worst of it is that because he practiced throwing with a heavier-than-normal weight, he imposed repetitive and excessive stress on his shoulder, elbow and wrist joints – all of which could've been avoided if he utilized a sensible approach to developing his strength by lifting weights and improving his skill by throwing a 15-ounce, prolate spheroid rather than a five-pound, hex-head dumbbell.

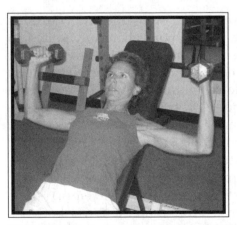

Figure 2.3: On occasion, you can supplement your program with some single-joint movements for direct stimulation.

This discussion is also applicable to the performance of high-impact plyometric drills. Jumping over boxes, bounding over cones and leaping from platforms of great heights are specific skills and unnecessary evils. If you're a basketball player who wants to become a better rebounder, you need to practice rebounding on a basketball court in game-like situations. Jumping over a box will not help you to learn sport-specific skills such as positioning your body to secure a rebound, boxing out an opposing player or reacting to the bounce of the ball off the backboard or rim. Jumping over a box will only help you to improve your skill at jumping over a box.

Not to belabor the point but here are two more examples: If you're a sprinter who wants to get faster, you need to practice sprinting the intended distances as fast as possible; if you're a soccer player who wants to get better at dribbling a soccer ball, you need to practice dribbling a soccer ball.

One other point: Practice makes perfect . . . but only if the practice is perfect. Translation: If you practice with poor technique then you'll learn how to do the skill with poor technique.

Athletes should practice all of their skills with proper technique and regulation equipment (not equipment that's heavier – or lighter – than normal); otherwise, all that they're doing is forcing their neuromuscular systems to learn a new skill — a skill that won't be used in competition. The best way for athletes to become better at a skill is to practice the intended skill. And athletes who become stronger will increase their potential to become better.

Many injuries occur from trying to be "sport specific" whether it's using a dumbbell to mimic a skill in the weight room, doing a similar activity or using some type of overpriced, exotic gadget. Remember, performing a particular skill only makes you more proficient at that skill and nothing else.

Lifting Technique

One part of the equation for safe training is to avoid exercises in the weight room that are potentially harmful; a second part is to perform exercises in the weight room with proper technique. When you do an exercise with resistance – or any exercise for that matter – your muscles should do as much of the work as possible, not momentum. One way to define "momentum" is "mass in motion." So if a mass (a weight) is moving, then it has momentum. But using an excessive amount of momentum to lift a weight is greatly discouraged since it will be highly detrimental to your program.

Dan Riley, the Strength and Conditioning Coach of the Houston Texans, explains that the raising and lowering of a weight shouldn't be a "throw up and fall down." Instead, it should be done in a smooth, controlled manner through a full range of motion (or a range of motion that's orthopedically acceptable for you). When a repetition is performed in a deliberate manner – meaning that it's done without an excessive amount of momentum – the targeted muscle is continuously loaded. As a result, there's a greater potential for the muscle to gain strength throughout its entire range of motion – and with a much lower potential for injury.

For a muscle to receive the greatest benefits and to reduce the risk of injury, there are four aspects of a repetition that you must consider:

1. The start/finish position.

2. The concentric or positive phase. (When you raise the weight.)

3. The mid-range or contracted position.

4. The eccentric or negative phase. (When you lower the weight.)

At the start of every repetition, you should use great care to "squeeze off" the weight under control using a smooth and deliberate movement. You shouldn't jerk, heave, bounce, snap or throw the weight. This only increases the involvement of momentum, reduces the emphasis on the targeted muscle and puts undue stress on the joints and soft tissues at both the start/finish position as well as the mid-range position. If you do an abrupt movement at the beginning of the repetition, the end result is usually a sudden "slam-on-the-brakes" arrival at the mid-range position. This puts an enormous and undesirable amount of torque on the joints and the muscle. Frequently, this "throw up" of the weight is followed by a quick and haphazard "fall down" of the weight.

Increasing the involvement of momentum is often done intentionally in order to bounce or "throw up" the weight back to the mid-range position. And then the vicious cycle continues. Obviously, this method doesn't effectively address the targeted muscle; rather, it serves only to reduce the effectiveness of the exercise, massage the ego since a heavier weight is used (basically under false pretenses) and takes a perilous step closer to an injury.

Let's take a look at the four-step process of executing a repetition in a safe, effective and efficient manner.

Step 1: Pause briefly in the start/finish position so that a minimum amount of momentum is used to initiate movement of the weight.

Step 2: Raise the weight in a deliberate manner in order to maintain a constant load on the targeted muscle. This should take at least two seconds to do.

Step 3: Pause briefly in the mid-range position. The pause isn't done for the purpose of relaxing. If anything, it's just the opposite: It's done to emphasize the targeted muscle and establish control to reduce stress on the joints and keep the targeted muscle loaded.

Step 4: Lower the weight in the same deliberate manner that was used to raise the weight. The lifter should ease out of the mid-range position to begin a slow and steady descent back to the start/finish position. This should take at least four seconds to do.

This safe, effective and efficient process is repeated for each subsequent repetition until the set is completed. These steps should comprise everyone's approach to performing quality repetitions for improved strength and fitness along with a reduced risk of injury.

The repetition speeds that have been noted for the raising and lowering of the weight are merely approximations. An appropriate speed of movement is dictated by several factors, including . . .

1. the exercise being performed and its range of motion. The overhead press has a much greater range of motion than the shrug. Therefore, it should take a little bit more time to do a repetition of the overhead press in comparison to the shrug.

2. your physical structure. In the same exercise, an individual with longer limbs has to move the weight a greater distance than an individual with shorter limbs. A good example is the bent-over row. Clearly, someone whose arms are 34 inches long must move the dumbbell farther than someone whose arms are 28 inches. Therefore, it should take a little bit more time to do a repetition in which the weight travels 34 inches in comparison to 28 inches.

3. your personal preferences. Some individuals simply prefer to do repetitions with certain speeds of movement whether it's raising the weight in two seconds and lowering it in four (a 2/4 speed) or raising the weight in 10 seconds and lowering it in five (a 10/5 speed).

So a good way to approach each exercise is to move the weight at the same controlled speed for all exercises and let the time take care of itself. The key points to remember are to (1) focus on proper technique using a controlled method that minimizes momentum; (2) keep a constant load on the targeted muscle; (3) avoid using "body English" so that the risk of injury is minimized and the involvement of the targeted muscle is maximized.

To make things perfectly clear, nowhere during the repetition should the load be removed from the targeted muscle.

You should never relax in the start/finish or mid-range positions, especially since this puts a tremendous amount of stress on the joints and allows the targeted muscle a chance to rest thereby reducing the effectiveness of the exercise.

> *"The object of a set is to stimulate as many muscle fibers as possible."*
> – Kim Wood,
> Strength Coach,
> Cincinnati Bengals
> (1975-2003)

Consider the supine (flat bench) press when the dumbbells are held near your chest in the start/finish position. By relaxing the targeted muscles (the chest, anterior deltoids and triceps), your joints (the shoulders, elbows and wrists) will absorb most of the stress. This reduces the effectiveness of the movement and places unnecessary stress on those joints. You must keep the muscle working – or "under load" – at all times through the entire range of motion for all repetitions until you complete the set. All of which is done with proper technique and control.

EFFECTIVENESS AND EFFICIENCY

As stated in the beginning of this chapter, there are many approaches that can be used to improve strength and fitness. Some are better than others because they're safer; some are better than others because they're effective and efficient. The best approach is one that combines safety, effectiveness and efficiency.

This type of approach is nothing new or groundbreaking. In fact, it has been around in one form or another for nearly 50 years. It was brought mainstream in the very early 1970s by Arthur Jones, the inventor of Nautilus® equipment. Jones was a man of deep thought. Among other things, he felt that an individual should be as strong and as fit as possible.

Intensity

Largely through trial and error, Jones determined that the safest, most efficient and most effective way to improve strength and fitness at the same time is to do approximately 10 - 12 exercises in each workout that address the entire body, perform one or two sets of each exercise to the point of muscular fatigue and complete the workout as quickly as possible (while maintaining good lifting technique, of course).

Not only has this been found to make an individual strong and fit but it also improves what Jones referred to as "metabolic conditioning." Simply put, metabolic conditioning is the ability to involve the musculoskeletal and cardiorespiratory systems simultaneously with intense workloads for a prescribed period of time. Essentially, it's doing an anaerobic activity (such as high-intensity strength training) in an aerobic environment (about 15 - 30 minutes of near continuous activity). And the only way to achieve this is to perform each exercise with a high level of intensity (or effort), meaning that each set is taken to the point of muscular fatigue while resting as briefly as possible between exercises/sets. Clearly, Arthur Jones was no dumbbell.

Exercise Sequence

Jones also suggested that the muscles should be worked in a descending order according to their size and strength output. In other words, you should work your muscles in this sequence: hips, legs (upper and lower), torso (chest, upper back and shoulders), arms (upper and lower) and mid-section (abdominals and lower back).

This order of exercise isn't etched in stone, however; it's merely a general guideline. Suppose that in your program, you wanted to include the shrug with dumbbells, it wouldn't be a bad idea to perform that exercise prior to those that fatigue the muscles of your hips, legs and lower back. The reason is that when you do exercises in the standing position, your lower body and lower back act as stabilizers. This is especially true when using heavy weights. As Dr. Leistner notes, "There is quite a bit of indirect work given to the muscles of the low back and hips as the body is held in proper position. The compressive forces that affect the spine are, in part, dissipated through the lower extremities, providing some reduction of the forces which must be borne by the lumbar spine components. In many instances, however, the lumbar spine is still exposed to a great deal of compressive force due to the amount of weight being used." In other words, your lower body and lower back may not be capable of supporting you properly if the muscles that affect those areas are fatigued. Plus, this may increase the risk of injury to your lower back.

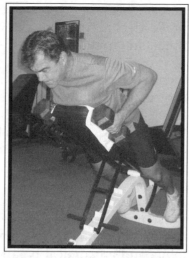

Figure 2.4: High-intensity training can improve strength and fitness and develop mental toughness.

Another reason why you might stray from the recommended largest-to-smallest sequence is if you want to prioritize a body part or particular exercise that's lagging in development. In this case, you can perform it first in your workout. This will allow you to target it when you're fresh.

Exercise Choices

By choosing one or two exercises to address each of the aforementioned muscles – either directly or indirectly – you have the makings for a well-rounded, comprehensive workout. A good rule of thumb is to select (1) one or two multiple-joint movements for your lower body such as the deadlift, squat or lunge; (2) two multiple-joint "pushing" movements for your torso such as the supine press, incline press, decline press or overhead press and (3) two multiple-joint "pulling" movements for your torso such as the bent-over row or bench row. On occasion, you can supplement your program with some single-joint movements for direct stimulation such as the lateral raise, bicep curl and tricep extension. (To avoid confusion, it's important to note that all muscles "pull" when they contract; however, muscle contractions cause joints to extend and flex which produce movements that can be described as either "pushing" or "pulling.")

Here, the key is to maintain balance in pushing/pulling movements as well as exercises that address the front/back of your body in order to provide structural integrity to your joints and anatomical balance to your muscles. Now, this doesn't mean that you have to perform exactly equal amounts of work for the front and back parts of your body in each training session. But over the course of a week, your choice of exercises should provide roughly an equal amount of emphasis on all of your major muscles. So, you can emphasize more pushing movements in your Monday workout, more pulling movements in your Wednesday workout and a more balanced routine of pushing and pulling movements in your Friday workout. The goal is to keep from becoming "lopsided" or imbalanced in your approach and physical structure.

The design of a workout can have almost an infinite number of possibilities. But a basic workout with dumbbells that covers your entire musculature might look like this (sets x repetitions):

Shrug - 1 x 12
Deadlift - 1 x 20
Seated Calf Raise - 1 x 15 (each leg)
Incline Press - 1 x 10
Bent-Over Row - 1 x 10 (each arm)
Overhead Press - 1 x 10
Bicep Curl - 1 x 10

Wrist Extension - 1 x 12 (each arm)
Side Bend - 1 x 12 (each side)

As you can see, all of the major muscles are being addressed in just nine exercises and only one all-out set is performed in this workout. Each set is taken to the point where another repetition cannot be performed with good form – where the working muscle fibers have been stimulated 100%. If each set is taken to this point of fatigue and the recovery between exercises is about 60 seconds or less, the level of effort is very high which produces a greater cardiorespiratory response than traditional workouts. It's not unusual for individuals to elevate their heart rates to 150 beats per minute or more by performing this type of metabolic work.

When done with a minute or less of recovery, this workout can be completed in less than 30 minutes. And who can't commit 30 minutes of their time, two or three times per week to improve their strength and fitness? If you're able to work with a high level of effort, you'll find your workouts to be short by necessity, yet highly effective. And that's why it's recommended that you train in this fashion a minimum of two but no more than three times per week.

This type of safe, effective and efficient approach has been dubbed "High-Intensity Training" or "HIT." It's used by numerous athletes at many major universities as well as professional teams in all of the major sports. However, you don't need to be an elite athlete to perform this kind of workout but you can certainly reap the same benefits when training with this level of effort and purpose.

A REAL-LIFE EXAMPLE

To define and illustrate the benefits of improved strength and fitness from workouts that emphasize metabolic conditioning, here's a real-life example that also shows how mental toughness is derived from such training:

Bob is a 53-year-old businessman who had never practiced any type of formalized strength training until he was

51 years of age. For 18 consecutive months, Bob trained religiously twice per week, performing total-body workouts that consisted of roughly eight sets for his entire workout. Bob performed each set to the point of muscular fatigue and his rest between exercises was no more than about 60 seconds. His workouts lasted roughly 22 minutes.

Bob is also an avid cyclist. On some of his non-training days, he bikes anywhere from 25 - 50 miles, while taking off select days to rest and recover so as not to overtrain. On occasion, Bob cycles a "century." As the name implies, this is a 100-mile bike ride that's taken along roads and winding streets against the elements. Bob prepares both physically and mentally to accomplish these particular rides. In his last century, he stated, "This was by far my best performance on the bike, bar none. Not only did I ride my best century but I also had my best average speed ever and I felt great after the ride. My recovery was great and my strength was incredible but at the 95th mile, I felt like I was losing it. My body was starting to shut down but it was the mental aspect of pushing for more in the weight room that allowed me to push on and get me to my destination. That's what put me over the top."

THE BOTTOM LINE

Being strong is important but being fit is of equal value. It doesn't matter much if you can lift heavy dumbbells but can't walk/run short distances or enjoy normal recreational activities because you aren't "in shape." Training with a high level of intensity while taking a minimum amount of recovery between exercises will enable you to get strong *and* fit in a safe, effective and efficient manner.

REFERENCES:

Leistner, K. 1985. Specificity. *The Steel Tip* 1 (2): 4.

_____. 1985. The press: seated or standing? *The Steel Tip* 1 (7): 6.

Mannie, K. 1997. That quick response to your athletes' training needs. *Coach and Athletic Director* 66 (10) 32-33.

Wolf, M. D. 1982. Muscles: structure, function, and control. In *Strength training by the experts, 2nd ed*, ed D. P. Riley, 27-40. West Point, NY: Leisure Press.

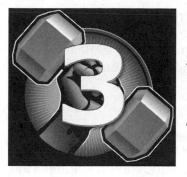

HARDEN YOUR HIPS AND LEGS

Because such a large amount of muscle mass is located below your waist, it's generally the most important region in the body. Therefore, a comprehensive strength-training workout must address the muscles of your hips and legs.

MUSCLES OF THE HIPS

Your hip region is made up of three main muscle groups: the gluteals, adductors and iliopsoas.

Gluteals

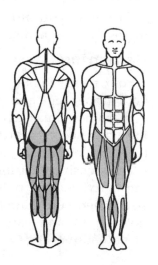

Your gluteals (or "glutes") are located on the back of your hips. They're composed of three primary muscles: the gluteus maximus, gluteus medius and gluteus minimus. The largest and strongest muscle in your body is your gluteus maximus (which forms your buttocks or "butt"). The main function of this muscle is hip extension (driving your upper legs backward). Your gluteus medius and gluteus minimus cause hip abduction (spreading your legs apart). Your gluteal muscles are involved significantly in walking, running, jumping and stairclimbing.

Adductors

Your adductor group is composed of five muscles that are found throughout your inner thigh. The muscles of your inner thigh are used during hip adduction (bringing your legs together).

Iliopsoas

The "iliopsoas" is actually a collective term for three muscles on the front of your hips: the iliacus, psoas major and psoas minor. The main function of the iliopsoas is hip flexion (bringing your knees to your chest). Your iliopsoas has a major role in many activities such as lifting your knees when walking, running and stairclimbing. The iliopsoas is sometimes considered with the muscles of the abdomen. Because of this, exercises for the iliopsoas are also discussed with those of the abdominals (Chapter 8).

MUSCLES OF THE UPPER LEGS

The two main muscle groups of your upper legs (or thighs) are the hamstrings and quadriceps.

Hamstrings

Your hamstrings (or "hams") are found on the back of your upper legs and actually include three muscles. Together, these muscles are involved in knee flexion (bringing your heels toward your buttocks) and hip extension (driving your upper legs backward). Your hamstrings are used extensively during virtually every running and jumping activity. One of the best reasons that you should strengthen your hamstrings is that they're quite susceptible to pulls and tears. Clearly, strong muscles on the back of your upper legs are necessary to counterbalance the powerful muscles on the front of your upper legs.

Quadriceps

Your quadriceps (or "quads") are the most important muscles on the front of your upper legs. As the name suggests, your quadriceps are made up of four muscles. The main function of your quadriceps is knee extension (straightening your legs). Your quadriceps are involved in all running, kicking and jumping skills.

MUSCLES OF THE LOWER LEGS

The calves and the "dorsi flexors" are the two major muscle groups in your lower legs.

Calves

Your calves are made up of two important muscles – the gastrocnemius (or "gastroc") and soleus – that are located on the back of your lower legs. These two muscles have a common tendon of insertion – the Achilles tendon – and are jointly referred to as the "triceps surae" or, more simply, the "gastroc-soleus." Your soleus actually resides underneath your gastrocnemius and is used primarily when you extendyour ankle while the angle between your upper and lower legs is about 90 degrees or less (such as in the seated position). The calves are involved in plantar flexion (extending your ankles or rising up on your toes). Your calves play a major role in running and jumping activities.

Dorsi Flexors

The front of your lower leg contains four muscles that are sometimes simply referred to as the "dorsi flexors." The largest of these muscles is the tibialis anterior. The dorsi flexors are primarily used in dorsi flexion (flexing your ankles). It's critical to strengthen your dorsi flexors as a safeguard against shin splints.

EXERCISES FOR THE HIPS AND LEGS

This chapter will describe and illustrate 11 exercises that

you can perform for your hip and leg muscles. These exercises are the deadlift, squat, ball squat, wall sit, lunge, step-up, hip abduction, hip flexion, seated calf raise, standing calf raise and dorsi flexion.

DEADLIFT

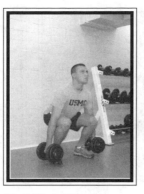 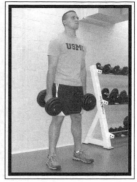

Start/Finish Position   *Mid-Range Position*

Muscles Influenced: gluteus maximus (buttocks), hamstrings, quadriceps and erector spinae (lower back)

Suggested Repetitions: 15 - 20

Start/Finish Position: Spread your feet slightly wider than shoulder-width apart and point them straight ahead. Lower yourself so that your upper legs are approximately parallel to the floor. Grasp a dumbbell with each hand. Flatten your back and look up slightly. Place most of your bodyweight on your heels. Straighten your arms and point your palms toward each other.

Performance Description: Stand upright until your legs and torso are almost completely straight. Pause briefly in this mid-range position (your legs and torso almost completely straight) and then lower your body under control to the start/finish position (your hips, legs and torso bent).

Training Tips:

- Avoid raising your hips too early as you perform this exercise.
- Exert force through your heels, not the balls of your feet.
- Avoid "locking" or "snapping" your knees in the mid-range position.
- Use wrist straps if you have difficulty in maintaining your grip on the dumbbells.
- Avoid this exercise if you have low-back pain, hyperextended elbows or an exceptionally long torso and/or legs.

SQUAT

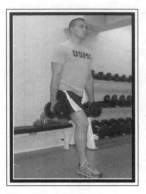 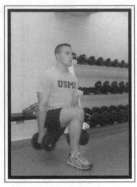

Start/Finish Position   *Mid-Range Position*

Muscles Influenced: gluteus maximus, hamstrings and quadriceps

Suggested Repetitions: 15 - 20

Start/Finish Position: Grasp a dumbbell with each hand. Position your right foot as described below in the training tips and point it straight ahead. Place your left lower leg on a bench (or a chair or stool). Straighten your right leg until it's almost completely extended. Place most of your bodyweight on your right heel. Straighten your arms and point your palms toward each other.

Performance Description: Lower yourself under control until your right upper leg is approximately parallel to the floor. Without bouncing, return to the start/finish position (your right leg almost completely straight). After performing a set with your right leg, repeat the exercise for the other side of your body.

Training Tips:

- Adjust the position of your forward foot so that your lower leg is perpendicular to the floor in the mid-range position.
- Exert force through your heel, not the ball of your foot.
- Avoid "locking" or "snapping" your knee in the start/finish position.
- Perform this exercise without the dumbbell if you cannot do 15 repetitions.

BALL SQUAT

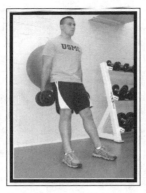 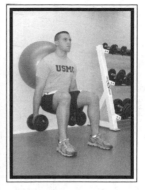

Start/Finish Position   Mid-Range Position

Muscles Influenced: gluteus maximus, hamstrings and quadriceps

Suggested Repetitions: 15 - 20

Start/Finish Position: Grasp a dumbbell with each hand. Position your heels a few feet in front of a smooth, unobstructed wall. Have a spotter or training partner place a stability ball between your lower back and the wall. Position your feet as described below in the training tips and spread them slightly wider than shoulder-width apart. Point your feet straight ahead. Straighten your legs until they're almost completely extended. Place most of your bodyweight on your heels. Straighten your arms and point your palms toward each other.

Performance Description: Lower yourself under control until your upper legs are approximately parallel to the floor. Without bouncing, return to the start/finish position (your legs almost completely straight).

Training Tips:

- Adjust the position of your feet so that your lower legs are perpendicular to the floor in the mid-range position.
- Exert force through your heels, not the balls of your feet.
- Avoid "locking" or "snapping" your knees in the start/finish position.
- Perform this exercise without the dumbbells if you cannot do 15 repetitions.

WALL SIT

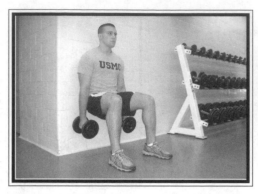

Start/Finish Position

Muscles Influenced: gluteus maximus, hamstrings and quadriceps

Suggested Time: 90 - 120 seconds

Start/Finish Position: Grasp a dumbbell with each hand. Position your torso flat against a smooth, unobstructed wall so that your upper legs are approximately parallel to the floor and your lower legs are perpendicular to the floor. Spread your feet slightly wider than shoulder-width apart and point them straight ahead. Place most of your bodyweight on your heels. Straighten your arms and point your palms toward each other.

Performance Description: Remain in the start/finish position for the suggested amount of time.

Training Tips:

- Exert force through your heels, not the balls of your feet.
- Perform this exercise without the dumbbells if you cannot do 90 seconds.

LUNGE

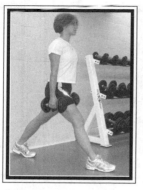 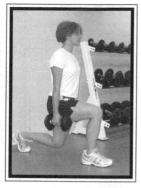

Start/Finish Position   Mid-Range Position

Muscles Influenced: gluteus maximus, hamstrings and quadriceps

Suggested Repetitions: 15 - 20

Start/Finish Position: Grasp a dumbbell with each hand. Step forward with your right foot and position your right lower leg so that it's perpendicular to the floor. Elevate your left heel off the floor. Point your feet straight ahead. Straighten your right leg until it's almost completely extended. Place most of your bodyweight on your right heel. Straighten your arms and point your palms toward each other.

Performance Description: Lower yourself under control until your right upper leg is approximately parallel to the floor. Without bouncing, return to the start/finish position (your right leg almost completely straight). After performing a set with your right leg, repeat the exercise for the other side of your body.

Training Tips:

• Exert force through your heel, not the ball of your foot.

• Avoid "locking" or "snapping" your knee in the start/finish position.

• Perform this exercise without the dumbbells if you cannot do 15 repetitions.

STEP-UP

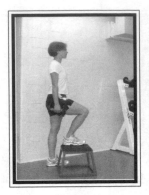 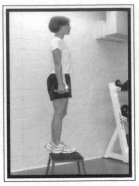

Start/Finish Position   Mid-Range Position

Muscles Influenced: gluteus maximus, hamstrings and quadriceps

Suggested Repetitions: 15 - 20

Start/Finish Position: Grasp a dumbbell with each hand. Place your right foot on a step that's about 18 - 24 inches high (or something similar that's stable). Position your right lower leg so that it's perpendicular to the floor. Straighten your left leg. Point your feet straight ahead. Place most of your bodyweight on your right heel. Straighten your arms and point your palms toward each other.

Performance Description: Stand up until your leg is almost completely straight. Pause briefly in this mid-range position (your leg almost completely straight) and then lower your body under control to the start/finish position (your leg bent). After performing a set with your right leg, repeat the exercise for the other side of your body.

Training Tips:

- Avoid using your non-exercising leg to assist your exercising leg.
- Exert force through your heel, not the ball of your foot.
- Avoid "locking" or "snapping" your knee in the mid-range position.
- Perform this exercise without the dumbbells if you cannot do 15 repetitions.

HIP ABDUCTION

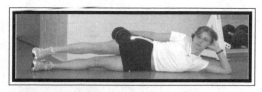

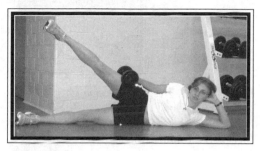

Start/Finish Position

Mid-Range Position

Muscle Influenced: gluteus medius

Suggested Repetitions: 10 - 15

Start/Finish Position: Grasp a dumbbell with your right hand. Lie down on the floor on your left side, straighten your legs and point your right toes toward your right knee. Position the dumbbell on the side of your right upper leg and hold it in place. Place your left hand against the left side of your head to support it.

Performance Description: Raise your right leg as high as possible. Pause briefly in this mid-range position (your legs apart) and then lower your right leg under control to the start/finish position (your legs together). After performing a set with your right leg, repeat the exercise for the other side of your body (lying on your right side).

Training Tips:

• Avoid bending forward at the waist as you perform this exercise.

• Raise your leg as high as possible in the mid-range position of every repetition.

• Perform this exercise without the dumbbell if you cannot do 15 repetitions.

HIP FLEXION

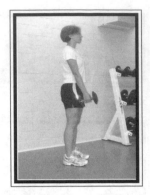 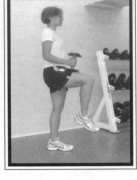

Start/Finish Position   *Mid-Range Position*

Muscle Influenced: iliopsoas (hip flexors)

Suggested Repetitions: 10 - 15

Start/Finish Position: Grasp a dumbbell with your right hand. Spread your feet about shoulder-width apart and point them straight ahead. Straighten your legs. Position the dumbbell on the top of your right upper leg and hold it in place.

Performance Description: Raise your right knee as high as possible. Pause briefly in this mid-range position (your leg bent) and then lower your leg under control to the start/finish position (your leg straight). After performing a set with your right leg, repeat the exercise for the other side of your body.

Training Tips:

- Avoid bending forward at the waist as you perform this exercise.
- Raise your knee as high as possible in the mid-range position of every repetition.

SEATED CALF RAISE

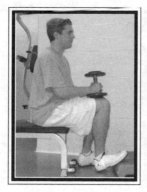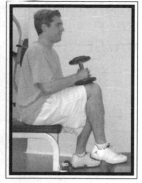

Start/Finish Position   Mid-Range Position

Muscles Influenced: gastrocnemius (calves) and soleus (calves)

Suggested Repetitions: 10 - 15

Start/Finish Position: Grasp a dumbbell with your right hand. Sit down near the end of a bench (or a chair or stool). Place the ball of your right foot on the edge of a step (or something similar that's stable) and lower your heel. Position the dumbbell on the top of your right upper leg and hold it in place.

Performance Description: Rise up onto your toes as high as possible. Pause briefly in this mid-range position (your ankle extended) and then lower your leg under control to the start/finish position (your heel near the floor). After performing a set with your right ankle, repeat the exercise for the other side of your body.

Training Tips:

• Avoid this exercise if you have shin splints.

STANDING CALF RAISE

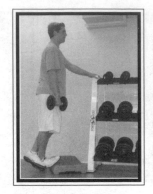 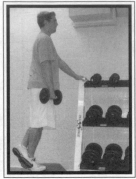

Start/Finish Position   Mid-Range Position

Muscles Influenced: gastrocnemius (calves)

Suggested Repetitions: 10 - 15

Start/Finish Position: Grasp a dumbbell with your right hand. Place
the ball of your right foot on the edge of a step (or something
similar that's stable) and lower your heel. Hold onto the railing
(or something similar) to maintain your balance. Straighten your
right leg until it's almost completely extended. Cross your left
foot behind your right foot. Straighten your right arm and point
your right hand toward your leg.

Performance Description: Keeping your right leg almost completely
extended, rise up onto your toes as high as possible. Pause briefly
in this mid-range position (your ankle extended) and then lower
your body under control to the start/finish position (your heel
near the floor). After performing a set with your right ankle, repeat the exercise for the other side of your body (holding the
dumbbell with your left hand).

Training Tips:

- Use a wrist strap if you have difficulty in maintaining a grip on
the dumbbell.
- Perform this exercise without the dumbbell if you cannot do 15
repetitions.
- Avoid this exercise if you have shin splints.

DORSI FLEXION

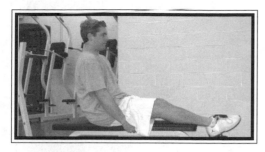

Start/Finish Position

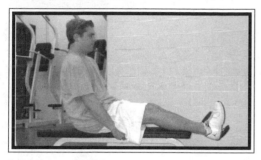

Mid-Range Position

Muscles Influenced: dorsi flexors

Suggested Repetitions: 10 - 15

Start/Finish Position: Grasp a dumbbell with your preferred hand. Sit down near the end of a bench and place the dumbbell between your feet. Slide your hips back so that your legs lie across the length of the pad. Position your heels slightly over the end of the pad and point your toes away from your body.

Performance Description: Keeping your legs flat on the pad, flex your ankles as much as possible. Pause briefly in this mid-range position (your ankles flexed) and then lower the dumbbell under control to the start/finish position (your ankles completely extended).

Training Tips:

• Avoid this exercise if you have shin splints.

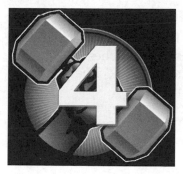

CHALLENGE YOUR CHEST

The chest area – along with the upper back and shoulders – is one of the major muscle groups in your torso.

MUSCLES OF THE CHEST

The main muscles that surround your chest area are the pectoralis major and pectoralis minor. The pectoralis major is thick, flat and fan-shaped and the most superficial muscle of your chest wall. The pectoralis minor is thin, flat and triangular and positioned beneath your pectoralis major. The "pecs" pull your upper arms across your body. Like most of the muscles in the torso, your chest is involved in throwing and pushing movements.

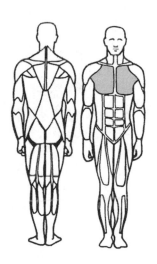

EXERCISES FOR THE CHEST

This chapter will describe and illustrate six exercises that you can perform for the muscles of your chest. The exercises are the supine press, incline press, decline press, supine fly, incline fly and decline fly.

SUPINE PRESS

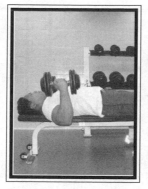 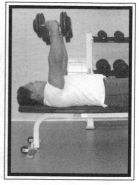

Start/Finish Position　　　*Mid-Range Position*

Muscles Influenced: chest, anterior deltoids and triceps

Suggested Repetitions: 6 - 12

Start/Finish Position: Grasp a dumbbell with each hand. Sit down near the end of a bench. Lie down on the bench and place your feet flat on the floor. Position the dumbbells on both sides of your torso so that your hands are even with your chest. Point your palms toward each other.

Performance Description: Push the dumbbells up until your arms are almost completely straight. Pause briefly in this mid-range position (your arms almost completely straight) and then lower the dumbbells under control to the start/finish position (your arms bent).

Training Tips:

- Keep your hips flat on the bench and your feet flat on the floor as you perform this exercise. Placing your feet on the end of the bench (or a chair or stool) will reduce the stress in your low-back region.

- Avoid "locking" or "snapping" your elbows in the mid-range position.

- Bring your hands closer together as you raise the dumbbells.

INCLINE PRESS

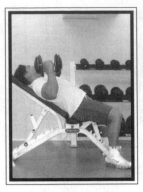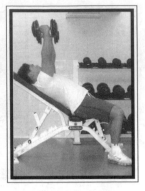

Start/Finish Position   Mid-Range Position

Muscles Influenced: chest (upper), anterior deltoids and triceps

Suggested Repetitions: 6 - 12

Start/Finish Position: Grasp a dumbbell with each hand. Sit down on the seat pad of an incline bench. Lie back against the bench and place your feet flat on the floor. Position the dumbbells on both sides of your torso so that your hands are even with your shoulders. Point your palms toward each other.

Performance Description: Push the dumbbells up until your arms are almost completely straight. Pause briefly in this mid-range position (your arms almost completely straight) and then lower the dumbbells under control to the start/finish position (your arms bent).

Training Tips:

- Keep your hips flat on the seat pad and your feet flat on the floor as you perform this exercise. Placing your feet on a chair or stool will reduce the stress in your low-back region.

- Avoid "locking" or "snapping" your elbows in the mid-range position.

- Bring your hands closer together as you raise the dumbbells.

DECLINE PRESS

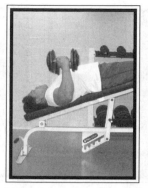 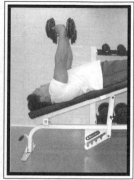

Start/Finish Position   Mid-Range Position

Muscles Influenced: chest (lower), anterior deltoid and triceps

Suggested Repetitions: 6 - 12

Start/Finish Position: Grasp a dumbbell with each hand. Sit down near the end of a decline bench. Place your lower legs behind the roller pads and lie down on the bench. Position the dumbbells on both sides of your torso so that your hands are even with your chest. Point your palms toward each other.

Performance Description: Push the dumbbells up until your arms are almost completely straight. Pause briefly in this mid-range position (your arms almost completely straight) and then lower the dumbbells under control to the start/finish position (your arms bent).

Training Tips:

- Keep your hips flat on the bench as you perform this exercise.
- Avoid "locking" or "snapping" your elbows in the mid-range position.
- Bring your hands closer together as you raise the dumbbells.

SUPINE FLY

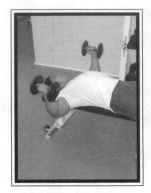 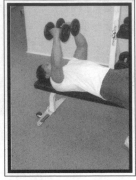

Start/Finish Position   Mid-Range Position

Muscles Influenced: chest and anterior deltoids

Suggested Repetitions: 6 - 12

Start/Finish Position: Grasp a dumbbell with each hand. Sit down near the end of a bench. Lie down on the bench and place your feet flat on the floor. Position the dumbbells on both sides of your torso so that your hands are even with your chest. Point your palms toward each other and move the dumbbells away from your chest until the angle between your upper and lower arms is about 90 degrees.

Performance Description: Keeping the same angle between your upper and lower arms, bring the dumbbells together above your chest. Pause briefly in this mid-range position (your arms close together) and then lower the dumbbells under control to the start/ finish position (your arms spread apart).

Training Tips:

- Maintain about a 90-degree angle between your upper and lower arms as you raise and lower the dumbbells. (Imagine that you're hugging a tree.)

- Keep your hips flat on the bench and your feet flat on the floor as you perform this exercise. Placing your feet on the end of the bench (or a chair or stool) will reduce the stress in your low-back region.

INCLINE FLY

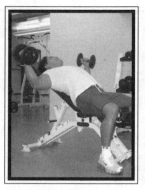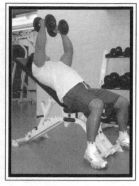

Start/Finish Position   *Mid-Range Position*

Muscles Influenced: chest (upper) and anterior deltoids

Suggested Repetitions: 6 - 12

Start/Finish Position: Grasp a dumbbell with each hand. Sit down on the seat pad of an incline bench. Lie back against the bench and place your feet flat on the floor. Position the dumbbells on both sides of your torso so that your hands are even with your shoulders. Point your palms toward each other and move the dumbbells away from your shoulders until the angle between your upper and lower arms is about 90 degrees.

Performance Description: Keeping the same angle between your upper and lower arms, bring the dumbbells together above your chest. Pause briefly in this mid-range position (your arms close together) and then lower the dumbbells under control to the start/finish position (your arms spread apart).

Training Tips:

* Maintain about a 90-degree angle between your upper and lower arms as you raise and lower the dumbbells. (Imagine that you're hugging a tree.)

* Keep your hips flat on the seat pad and your feet flat on the floor as you perform this exercise. Placing your feet on a chair or stool will reduce the stress in your low-back region.

DECLINE FLY

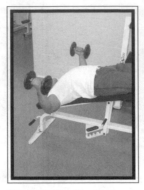
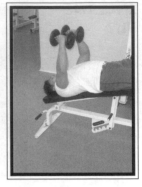

Start/Finish Position   Mid-Range Position

Muscles Influenced: chest (lower) and anterior deltoids

Suggested Repetitions: 6 - 12

Start/Finish Position: Grasp a dumbbell with each hand. Sit down near the end of a decline bench. Place your lower legs behind the roller pads and lie down on the bench. Position the dumbbells on both sides of your torso so that your hands are even with your chest. Point your palms toward each other and move the dumbbells away from your chest until the angle between your upper and lower arms is about 90 degrees.

Performance Description: Keeping the same angle between your upper and lower arms, bring the dumbbells together above your chest. Pause briefly in this mid-range position (your arms close together) and then lower the dumbbells under control to the start/ finish position (your arms spread apart).

Training Tips:

- Maintain about a 90-degree angle between your upper and lower arms as you raise and lower the dumbbells. (Imagine that you're hugging a tree.)
- Keep your hips flat on the bench as you perform this exercise.

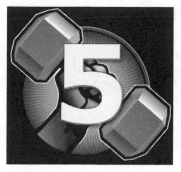

OVERHAUL YOUR UPPER BACK

The upper back – along with the chest and shoulders – is one of the major muscle groups in your torso.

MUSCLES OF THE UPPER BACK

The latissimus dorsi is a long, broad muscle that comprises most of your upper back. As a matter of fact, the "lats" are the largest muscle in your torso. Its primary function is to pull your upper arms backward and downward. The muscle is particularly important in assorted pulling movements and climbing skills. In addition, developing the latissimus dorsi is necessary to provide muscular balance between your upper back and chest.

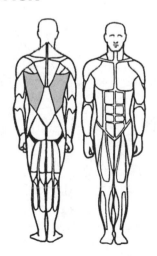

EXERCISES FOR THE UPPER BACK

This chapter will describe and illustrate three exercises that you can perform for the muscles of your upper back. The exercises are the bench row, bent-over row and pull-over.

BENCH ROW

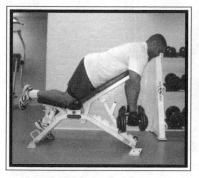 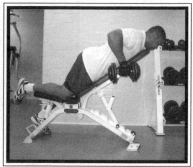

Start/Finish Position   *Mid-Range Position*

Muscles Influenced: upper back ("lats"), biceps and forearms

Suggested Repetitions: 6 - 12

Start/Finish Position: Grasp a dumbbell with each hand. Place one knee on the seat pad of an incline bench and the opposite foot on the floor. Lie forward against the bench and position the dumbbells below your torso. Straighten your arms and point your palms toward each other.

Performance Description: Keeping your elbows close to your torso, pull the dumbbells up to your shoulders. Pause briefly in this mid-range position (your arms bent) and then lower the dumbbells under control to the start/finish position (your arms straight).

Training Tips:

- Avoid throwing the dumbbells by using your legs or swinging your torso. Movement should only occur around your shoulder and elbow joints.

- Do this exercise with one limb at a time if you have a shoulder or an arm injury, a gross difference in the strength between your limbs or desire a training variation.

- Use wrist straps if you have difficulty in maintaining your grip on the dumbbells.

- Avoid this exercise if you have hyperextended elbows.

BENT-OVER ROW

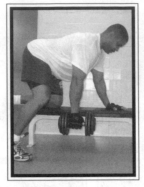 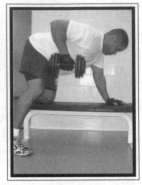

Start/Finish Position   Mid-Range Position

Muscles Influenced: upper back ("lats"), biceps and forearms

Suggested Repetitions: 6 - 12

Start/Finish Position: Grasp a dumbbell with your right hand. Place your left hand and left knee on a bench. Position your right foot on the floor at a comfortable distance from the bench. Straighten your right arm and point your palm toward the bench.

Performance Description: Keeping your elbow close to your torso, pull the dumbbell up to your right shoulder. Pause briefly in this mid-range position (your arm bent) and then lower the dumbbell under control to the start/finish position (your arm straight). After performing a set with your right arm, repeat the exercise for the other side of your body (with your right hand and right knee on the bench for support).

Training Tips:

- Avoid throwing the dumbbell by using your legs or rotating your torso. Movement should only occur around your shoulder and elbow joints.

- Use a wrist strap if you have difficulty in maintaining your grip on the dumbbell.

- Avoid this exercise if you have a hyperextended elbow.

PULLOVER

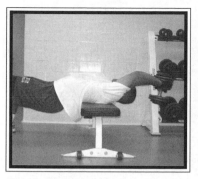 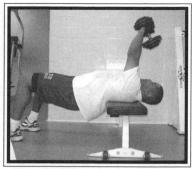

Start/Finish Position   *Mid-Range Position*

Muscles Influenced: upper back ("lats")

Suggested Repetitions: 6 - 12

Start/Finish Position: Grasp a dumbbell with both hands. Lie down across the middle of the bench. Position your shoulder blades such that your torso is perpendicular to the length of the bench and place your feet flat on the floor. Hold the dumbbell by placing your palms against the innermost plate (not the handle). Keep your arms relatively straight and lower the dumbbell toward the floor so that your elbows are near or slightly past your head.

Performance Description: Keeping your arms relatively straight, pull the dumbbell over your head until your arms are perpendicular to the floor. Pause briefly in this mid-range position (your arms perpendicular to the floor) and then lower the dumbbell under control to the start/finish position (your elbows near or slightly past your head).

Training Tips:

- Avoid this exercise if you have low-back pain or shoulder-impingement syndrome.

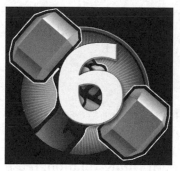

SHAPE YOUR SHOULDERS

The shoulders – along with the chest and upper back – are one of the major muscle groups in your torso.

MUSCLES OF THE SHOULDERS

Your shoulders are made up of 11 muscles. The primary muscles are the deltoids, the so-called "rotator cuff" and the trapezius.

Deltoids

The most important muscles in your shoulders are the deltoids. Your "delts" are actually composed of three separate parts (or "heads"). The anterior deltoid is found on the front of your shoulder and is used to raise your upper arm forward; the middle deltoid is located on the side of your shoul-

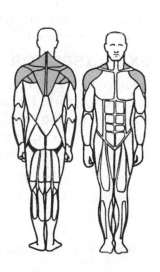

der and is used to raise your upper arm sideways; and the posterior deltoid is found on the back of your shoulder and is used to draw your upper arm backward.

Rotator Cuff

Several other deep muscles of the shoulder are sometimes referred to as the "internal rotators" (the subscapularis and teres major) and the "external rotators" (the infraspinatus and teres minor). In addition to performing rotation, these muscles are also largely responsible for maintaining the integrity of your shoulder joint and in preventing shoulder impingement. Along with the muscles of the chest, strong shoulders are a vital part of throwing skills and pushing movements.

Trapezius

The trapezius is a kite-shaped (or trapezoid-shaped) muscle that covers the uppermost region of your back and the posterior section of your neck. The primary functions of your "traps" are shoulder elevation (shrugging your shoulders as if to say, "I don't know"), scapulae adduction ("pinching" your shoulder blades together) and neck extension (bringing your head backward). The trapezius is often considered part of the neck musculature.

EXERCISES FOR THE SHOULDERS

This chapter will describe and illustrate 10 exercises that you can perform for the muscles of your shoulders. These exercises are the overhead press, lateral raise, front raise, bent-over raise, internal rotation, external rotation, upright row, shrug, bench shrug and scapula retraction.

OVERHEAD PRESS

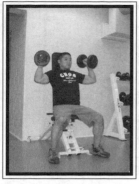 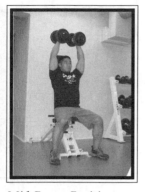

Start/Finish Position   Mid-Range Position

Muscles Influenced: anterior deltoids and triceps

Suggested Repetitions: 6 - 12

Start/Finish Position: Grasp a dumbbell with each hand. Sit down on the seat pad of a bench. Lie back against the bench (if it has a back pad) and place your feet flat on the floor. Position the dumbbells on both sides of your torso so that your hands are even with your shoulders. Point your palms toward each other.

Performance Description: Push the dumbbells up until your arms are almost completely straight. Pause briefly in this mid-range position (your arms almost completely straight) and then lower the dumbbells under control to the start/finish position (your arms bent).

Training Tips:

- Keep your hips flat on the seat pad and your feet flat on the floor as you perform this exercise. Placing your feet on a chair or stool will reduce the stress in your low-back region.

- Avoid "locking" or "snapping" your elbows in the mid-range position.

- Do this exercise with one limb at a time if you have a shoulder or an arm injury, a gross difference in the strength between your limbs or desire a training variation.

- Avoid this exercise if you have shoulder-impingement syndrome or low-back pain.

LATERAL RAISE

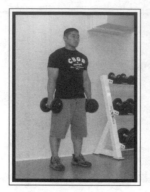 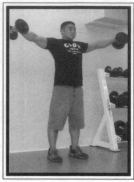

Start/Finish Position   Mid-Range Position

Muscles Influenced: middle deltoids and trapezius (upper)

Suggested Repetitions: 6 - 12

Start/Finish Position: Grasp a dumbbell with each hand. Position the dumbbells against the sides of your upper legs with your palms facing each other. Straighten your arms and spread your feet about shoulder-width apart.

Performance Description: Keeping your arms fairly straight, raise the dumbbells sideways until your arms are parallel to the floor. Pause briefly in this mid-range position (your arms parallel to the floor) and then lower the dumbbells under control to the start/finish position (your arms at your sides).

Training Tips:

- Avoid throwing the dumbbells by using your legs or swinging your torso. Movement should only occur around your shoulder joints.

- Raise your arms only to the point at which they're parallel to the floor.

- Do this exercise with one limb at a time if you have a shoulder or an arm injury, a gross difference in the strength between your limbs or desire a training variation.

FRONT RAISE

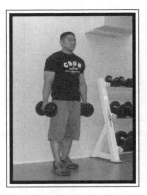 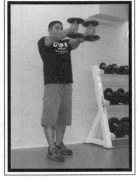

Start/Finish Position   Mid-Range Position

Muscle Influenced: anterior deltoids

Suggested Repetitions: 6 - 12

Start/Finish Position: Grasp a dumbbell with each hand. Hold the dumbbells against the sides of your upper legs with your palms facing each other. Straighten your arms and place one foot slightly in front of the other.

Performance Description: Keeping your arms fairly straight, raise the dumbbells forward until your arms are parallel to the floor. Pause briefly in this mid-range position (your arms parallel to the floor) and then lower the dumbbells under control to the start/finish position (your arms at your sides).

Training Tips:

- Avoid throwing the dumbbells by using your legs or swinging your torso. Movement should only occur around your shoulder joints.

- Raise your arms only to the point at which they're parallel to the floor.

- Do this exercise with one limb at a time if you have a shoulder or an arm injury, a gross difference in the strength between your limbs or desire a training variation.

BENT-OVER RAISE

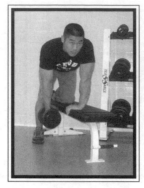 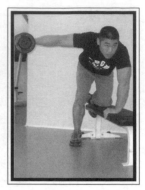

Start/Finish Position   Mid-Range Position

Muscle Influenced: posterior deltoid and trapezius (middle)

Suggested Repetitions: 6 - 12

Start/Finish Position: Grasp a dumbbell with your right hand. Place your left hand and left knee on a bench. Position your right foot on the floor at a comfortable distance from the bench. Straighten your right arm. Point your right palm toward the bench.

Performance Description: Keeping your arm fairly straight and perpendicular to your torso, raise the dumbbell sideways until your arm is parallel to the floor. Pause briefly in this mid-range position (your arm parallel to the floor) and then lower the dumbbell under control to the start/finish position (your arm near the bench). After performing a set with your right arm, repeat the exercise for the other side of your body (with your right hand and right knee on the bench for support).

Training Tips:

- Avoid throwing the dumbbell by using your legs or rotating your torso. Movement should only occur around your shoulder joint.
- Raise your arm only to the point at which it's parallel to the floor.

INTERNAL ROTATION

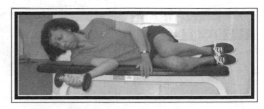

Start/Finish Position

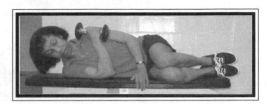

Mid-Range Position

Muscles Influenced: internal rotators

Suggested Repetitions: 6 - 12

Start/Finish Position: Grasp a dumbbell with your right hand. Lie down on a bench on your right side and draw your knees toward your torso. Position your right elbow just in front of your torso and bend your right arm so that the angle between your upper and lower arms is about 90 degrees. Point your right palm upward.

Performance Description: Keeping the same angle between your upper and lower arms, pull the dumbbell to your left shoulder. Pause briefly in this mid-range position (your hand near your shoulder) and then lower the dumbbell under control to the start/finish position (your hand away from your shoulder). After performing a set with your right arm, repeat the exercise for the other side of your body (while lying on your left side).

Training Tips:

- Avoid throwing the dumbbell by rotating your torso. Movement should only occur around your shoulder joint.

- Refrain from lying directly on your upper arm as you perform this exercise.

- Do this exercise on a bench (instead of the floor) to increase your range of motion and permit a greater stretch.

EXTERNAL ROTATION

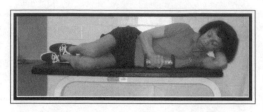

Start/Finish Position

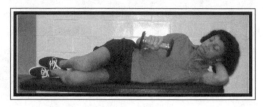

Mid-Range Position

Muscles Influenced: external rotators

Suggested Repetitions: 6 - 12

Start/Finish Position: Grasp a dumbbell with your right hand. Lie down on a bench on your left side and draw your knees toward your torso. Position your left arm just in front of your torso and lean back slightly. Keep your right elbow against your side and bend your right arm so that the angle between your upper and lower arms is about 90 degrees. Point your right palm downward.

Performance Description: Keeping the same angle between your upper and lower arms, raise the dumbbell as high as possible. Pause briefly in this mid-range position (your hand away from your mid-section) and then lower the dumbbell under control to the start/finish position (your hand near your mid-section). After performing a set with your right arm, repeat the exercise for the other side of your body (while lying on your right side).

Training Tips:

- Avoid throwing the dumbbell by rotating your torso. Movement should only occur around your shoulder joint.
- Do this exercise on a bench (instead of the floor) to increase your range of motion and permit a greater stretch.

UPRIGHT ROW

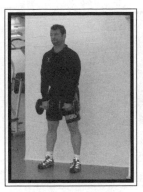 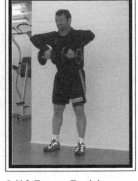

Start/Finish Position   *Mid-Range Position*

Muscles Influenced: trapezius (upper), biceps and forearms

Suggested Repetitions: 6 - 12

Start/Finish Position: Grasp a dumbbell with each hand. Position the dumbbells against the front of your upper legs with your palms facing your thighs. Straighten your arms and spread your feet about shoulder-width apart.

Performance Description: Pull the dumbbells up until your hands are just below your chin. Pause briefly in this mid-range position (your arms bent) and then lower the dumbbells under control to the start/finish position (your arms straight).

Training Tips:

- Avoid throwing the dumbbells by using your legs or swinging your torso. Movement should only occur around your shoulder and elbow joints.

- Keep the dumbbells close to your body as you perform this exercise.

- Use wrist straps if you have difficulty in maintaining your grip on the dumbbells.

- Avoid this exercise if you have low-back pain, hyperextended elbows or shoulder-impingement syndrome. (Raising the dumbbells to the lower part of your chest rather than to the upper part of it will reduce the stress on an impinged shoulder.)

SHRUG

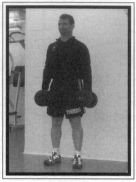

Start/Finish Position   Mid-Range Position

Muscle Influenced: trapezius (upper)

Suggested Repetitions: 8 - 12

Start/Finish Position: Grasp a dumbbell with each hand. Position the dumbbells against the sides of your upper legs with your palms facing each other. Straighten your arms and spread your feet about shoulder-width apart.

Performance Description: Keeping your arms fairly straight, pull the dumbbells up as high as possible. Pause briefly in this mid-range position (your shoulders near your ears) and then lower the dumbbells under control to the start/finish position (your shoulders away from your ears).

Training Tips:

- Refrain from "rolling" your shoulders as you perform this exercise.

- Avoid throwing the dumbbells by using your legs or swinging your torso. Movement should only occur around your shoulder joints.

- Do this exercise with one limb at a time if you have a shoulder or an arm injury, a gross difference in the strength between your limbs or desire a training variation.

- Use wrist straps if you have difficulty in maintaining your grip on the dumbbells.

- Avoid this exercise if you have low-back pain or hyperextended elbows.

BENCH SHRUG

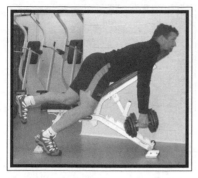 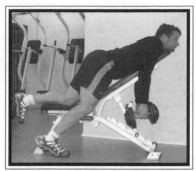

Start/Finish Position   Mid-Range Position

Muscle Influenced: trapezius (upper)

Suggested Repetitions: 8 - 12

Start/Finish Position: Grasp a dumbbell with each hand. Place one knee on the seat pad of an incline bench and the opposite foot on the floor. Lie forward against the bench and position the dumbbells below your torso. Straighten your arms and point your palms toward each other.

Performance Description: Keeping your arms fairly straight, pull the dumbbells up as high as possible. Pause briefly in this mid-range position (your shoulders near your ears) and then lower the dumbbells under control to the start/finish position (your shoulders away from your ears).

Training Tips:

- Refrain from "rolling" your shoulders as you perform this exercise.
- Avoid throwing the dumbbells by using your legs or swinging your torso. Movement should only occur around your shoulder joints.
- Do this exercise with one limb at a time if you have a shoulder or an arm injury, a gross difference in the strength between your limbs or desire a training variation.
- Use wrist straps if you have difficulty in maintaining your grip on the dumbbells.
- Avoid this exercise if you have hyperextended elbows.

SCAPULA RETRACTION

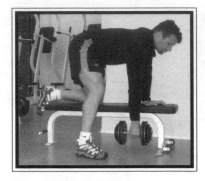
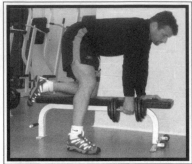

Start/Finish Position   Mid-Range Position

Muscles Influenced: trapezius (middle)

Suggested Repetitions: 8 - 12

Start/Finish Position: Grasp a dumbbell with your right hand. Place your left hand and left knee on a bench. Position your right foot on the floor at a comfortable distance from the bench. Straighten your right arm. Point your right palm toward the bench.

Performance Description: Keeping your arm fairly straight, pull the dumbbell up as high as possible. Pause briefly in this mid-range position (your shoulder near your ear) and then lower the dumbbell under control to the start/finish position (your shoulder away from your ear). After performing a set with your right arm, repeat the exercise for the other side of your body (with your right hand and right knee on the bench for support).

Training Tips:

- Avoid throwing the dumbbell by using your legs or rotating your torso. Movement should only occur around your shoulder joint.
- Use a wrist strap if you have difficulty in maintaining your grip on the dumbbell.
- Avoid this exercise if you have a hyperextended elbow.

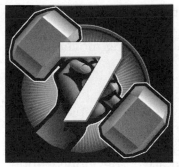

IMPROVE YOUR ARMS

Because your arms contain a relatively small amount of muscle mass, they're regarded as the "weak links" in multiple-joint movements for your torso. Therefore, it's critical for you to exercise these smaller, weaker muscles in order to strengthen the weak link.

MUSCLES OF THE UPPER ARMS

The two main muscles of your upper arms are the biceps and triceps.

Biceps

The prominent muscle that's located on the front of your upper arm is technically known as the "biceps brachii." As the name suggests, the biceps have two separate parts (or "heads"). The separation can sometimes be seen as a groove on a well-developed upper arm when the biceps are fully contracted. The pri-

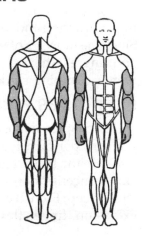

mary function of your biceps is elbow flexion (bending your arms). Your biceps assist the muscles of your torso – especially your "lats" – in pulling and climbing movements.

Triceps

The prominent muscle that's located on the back of your upper arm is technically known as the "triceps brachii." As the name suggests, the triceps have three distinct heads: the long, lateral and medial. These three heads produce a horseshoe-shaped appearance on a well-developed upper arm when the triceps are fully contracted. The primary function of your triceps is elbow extension (straightening your arms). Your triceps assist the muscles of your torso in pushing and throwing movements.

MUSCLES OF THE LOWER ARMS

The forearms are the major muscles in your lower arms.

Forearms

Amazingly as it may seem, each one of your forearms is made up of 19 different muscles. These muscles may be divided into two groups on the basis of their position and function. The anterior group on the front of your forearm causes wrist flexion (flexing your wrist) and pronation (turning your palm downward); the posterior group on the back of your forearm causes wrist extension (extending your wrist) and supination (turning your palm upward). Since the muscles of your forearms affect your wrists, hands and fingers, they're extremely important in pulling movements, climbing skills and tasks that involve gripping.

EXERCISES FOR THE ARMS

This chapter will describe and illustrate 14 exercises that you can perform for the muscles of your arms. The exercises are the bicep curl, hammer curl, reverse curl, preacher curl, concentration curl, tricep extension, cross tricep, incline tricep, French curl, tricep kickback, wrist flexion, wrist extension, finger flexion and pinch grip.

BICEP CURL

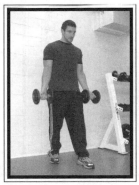

Start/Finish Position   Mid-Range Position

Muscles Influenced: biceps and forearms

Suggested Repetitions: 6 - 12

Start/Finish Position: Grasp a dumbbell with each hand. Position the dumbbells near the sides of your upper legs with your palms facing forward. Straighten your arms and place one foot slightly in front of the other.

Performance Description: Keeping your upper arms against the sides of your torso, pull the dumbbells up to your shoulders. Pause briefly in this mid-range position (your arms bent) and then lower the dumbbells under control to the start/finish position (your arms straight).

Training Tips:

- Avoid throwing the dumbbells by using your legs or swinging your torso. Movement should only occur around your elbow joints.

- Do this exercise with one limb at a time if you have an arm injury, a gross difference in the strength between your limbs or desire a training variation.

- Avoid this exercise if you have hyperextended elbows.

HAMMER CURL

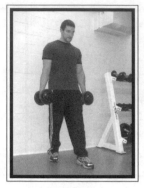 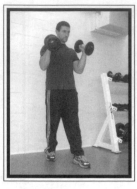

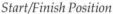

Start/Finish Position   *Mid-Range Position*

Muscles Influenced: biceps and forearms

Suggested Repetitions: 6 - 12

Start/Finish Position: Grasp a dumbbell with each hand. Position the dumbbells near the sides of your upper legs with your palms each other. Straighten your arms and place one foot slightly in front of the other.

Performance Description: Keeping your upper arms against the sides of your torso, pull the dumbbells up to your shoulders. Pause briefly in this mid-range position (your arms bent) and then lower the dumbbells under control to the start/finish position (your arms straight).

Training Tips:

- Avoid throwing the dumbbells by using your legs or swinging your torso. Movement should only occur around your elbow joints.

- Do this exercise with one limb at a time if you have an arm injury, a gross difference in the strength between your limbs or desire a training variation.

- Avoid this exercise if you have hyperextended elbows.

REVERSE CURL

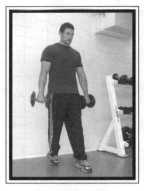 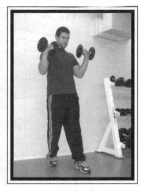

Start/Finish Position   *Mid-Range Position*

Muscles Influenced: biceps and forearms

Suggested Repetitions: 6 - 12

Start/Finish Position: Grasp a dumbbell with each hand. Position the dumbbells near the sides of your upper legs with your palms facing backward. Straighten your arms and place one foot slightly in front of the other.

Performance Description: Keeping your upper arms against the sides of your torso, pull the dumbbells up to your shoulders. Pause briefly in this mid-range position (your arms bent) and then lower the dumbbells under control to the start/finish position (your arms straight).

Training Tips:

- Avoid throwing the dumbbells by using your legs or swinging your torso. Movement should only occur around your elbow joints.

- Do this exercise with one limb at a time if you have an arm injury, a gross difference in the strength between your limbs or desire a training variation.

- Avoid this exercise if you have hyperextended elbows.

PREACHER CURL

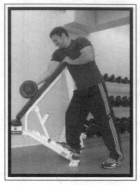
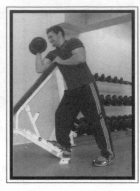

Start/Finish Position   Mid-Range Position

Muscles Influenced: biceps and forearms

Suggested Repetitions: 6 - 12

Start/Finish Position: Grasp a dumbbell with your right hand. Step behind the bench and place the back of your right upper arm on the pad. Straighten your right arm and place one foot slightly in front of the other. Place your left hand on your left hip or on the side of the bench. Point your right palm upward.

Performance Description: Keeping your upper arm against the pad, pull the dumbbell up to your right shoulder. Pause briefly in this mid-range position (your arm bent) and then lower the dumbbell under control to the start/finish position (your arm straight). After performing a set with your right arm, repeat the exercise for the other side of your body.

Training Tips:

• Avoid throwing the weight by using your legs or swinging your torso. Movement should only occur around your elbow joint.

• Avoid this exercise if you have a hyperextended elbow.

CONCENTRATION CURL

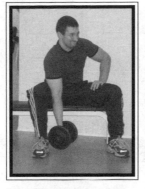 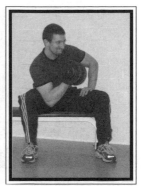

Start/Finish Position   *Mid-Range Position*

Muscles Influenced: biceps and forearm

Suggested Repetitions: 6 - 12

Start/Finish Position: Grasp a dumbbell with your right hand. Sit down near the end of a bench. Place the back of your right upper arm against the inside of your right upper leg. Straighten your right arm and place your feet flat on the floor. Place your left hand or lower arm on top of your left upper leg. Point your right palm away from your right leg.

Performance Description: Keeping your upper arm against the inside of your upper leg, pull the dumbbell up to your right shoulder. Pause briefly in this mid-range position (your arm bent) and then lower the dumbbell under control to the start/finish position (your arm straight). After performing a set with your right arm, repeat the exercise for the other side of your body.

Training Tips:

- Avoid throwing the weight by using your legs or swinging your torso. Movement should only occur around your elbow joint.

- Avoid this exercise if you have a hyperextended elbow.

TRICEP EXTENSION

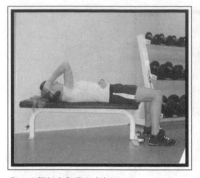
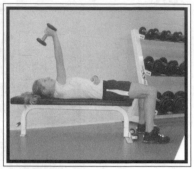

Start/Finish Position   *Mid-Range Position*

Muscle Influenced: triceps

Suggested Repetitions: 6 - 12

Start/Finish Position: Grasp a dumbbell with your right hand. Sit down near the end of a bench. Lie down on the bench and place your feet flat on the floor. Position your right upper arm so that it's approximately perpendicular to the floor and place the dumbbell near your right shoulder. Position your left lower arm across your mid-section. Point your right palm toward the right side of your head.

Performance Description: Keeping your upper arm perpendicular to the floor, straighten your arm. Pause briefly in this mid-range position (your arm straight) and then lower the dumbbell under control to the start/finish position (your arm bent). After performing a set with your right arm, repeat the exercise for the other side of your body.

Training Tips:

- Keep your hips flat on the bench and your feet flat on the floor as you perform this exercise. Placing your feet on the end of the bench (or a chair or stool) will reduce the stress in your low-back region.

- Avoid this exercise if you have shoulder-impingement syndrome.

CROSS TRICEP

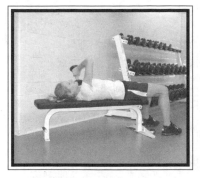 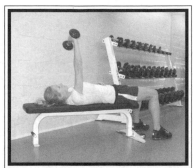

Start/Finish Position   Mid-Range Position

Muscle Influenced: triceps

Suggested Repetitions: 6 - 12

Start/Finish Position: Grasp a dumbbell with your right hand. Sit down near the end of a bench. Lie down on the bench and place your feet flat on the floor. Position your right upper arm so that it's approximately perpendicular to the floor and place the dumbbell near your left shoulder. Position your left lower arm across your mid-section. Point your right palm toward your left knee.

Performance Description: Keeping your upper arm perpendicular to the floor, straighten your arm. Pause briefly in this mid-range position (your arm straight) and then lower the dumbbell under control to the start/finish position (your arm bent). After performing a set with your right arm, repeat the exercise for the other side of your body.

Training Tips:

• Keep your hips flat on the bench and your feet flat on the floor as you perform this exercise. Placing your feet on the end of the bench (or a chair or stool) will reduce the stress in your low-back region.

• Avoid this exercise if you have shoulder-impingement syndrome.

INCLINE TRICEP

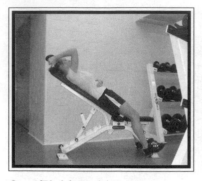

Start/Finish Position

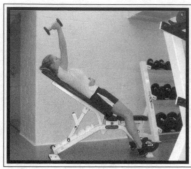

Mid-Range Position

Muscle Influenced: triceps

Suggested Repetitions: 6 - 12

Start/Finish Position: Grasp a dumbbell with your right hand. Straddle the seat pad of a bench but don't sit down. Lie back against the bench and place your feet flat on the floor. Position your right upper arm so that it's approximately perpendicular to the floor and place the dumbbell near your right shoulder. Position your left lower arm across your mid-section. Point your right palm toward the right side of your head.

Performance Description: Keeping your upper arm perpendicular to the floor, straighten your arm. Pause briefly in this mid-range position (your arm straight) and then lower the dumbbell under control to the start/finish position (your arm bent). After performing a set with your right arm, repeat the exercise for the other side of your body.

Training Tips:

- Keep your hips and torso against the bench as you perform this exercise. Movement should only occur around your elbow joint.
- Avoid this exercise if you have shoulder-impingement syndrome.

FRENCH CURL

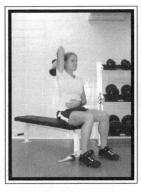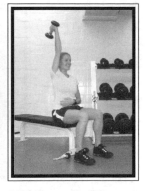

Start/Finish Position   Mid-Range Position

Muscle Influenced: triceps

Suggested Repetitions: 6 - 12

Start/Finish Position: Grasp a dumbbell with your right hand. Sit down near the end of a bench. Place your feet flat on the floor. Position your right upper arm so that it's approximately perpendicular to the floor and place the dumbbell behind your head near the base of your neck. Position your left lower arm across your mid-section. Point your right palm toward the back of your head.

Performance Description: Keeping your upper arm perpendicular to the floor, straighten your arm. Pause briefly in this mid-range position (your arm straight) and then lower the dumbbell under control to the start/finish position (your arm bent). After performing a set with your right arm, repeat the exercise for the other side of your body.

Training Tips:

- Avoid swinging your torso as you perform this exercise. Movement should only occur around your elbow joint.
- Avoid this exercise if you have shoulder-impingement syndrome.

TRICEP KICKBACK

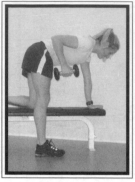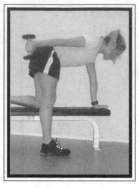

Start/Finish Position   Mid-Range Position

Muscle Influenced: triceps

Suggested Repetitions: 6 - 12

Start/Finish Position: Grasp a dumbbell with your right hand. Place your left hand and left knee on a bench. Position your right foot on the floor at a comfortable distance from the bench. Position your right upper arm against the right side of your torso and allow your right lower arm to hang straight down. Point your right palm toward the bench.

Performance Description: Keeping your upper arm against the side of your torso, straighten your arm. Pause briefly in this mid-range position (your arm straight) and then lower the dumbbell under control to the start/finish position (your arm bent). After performing a set with your right arm, repeat the exercise for the other side of your body (with your right hand and right knee on the bench for support).

Training Tips:

• Avoid throwing the dumbbell by using your legs or rotating your torso. Movement should only occur around your elbow joint.

WRIST FLEXION

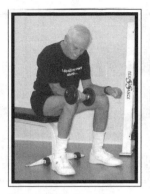
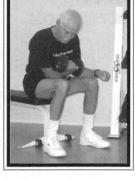

Start/Finish Position   Mid-Range Position

Muscles Influenced: wrist flexors

Suggested Repetitions: 8 - 12

Start/Finish Position: Grasp a dumbbell with your right hand. Sit down near the end of a bench (or a chair or stool) and place the back of your right forearm directly over your right upper leg so that your palm is facing up. Place your thumb underneath the handle alongside your fingers. Position your right wrist over your right kneecap. Lean forward slightly so that the angle between your upper and lower arms is about 90 degrees or less.

Performance Description: Pull the dumbbell up as high as possible by bending your wrist. Pause briefly in this mid-range position (your hand up) and then lower the dumbbell under control to the start/finish position (your hand down). After performing a set with your right arm, repeat the exercise for the other side of your body

Training Tips:

- Keep your forearm directly over your upper leg throughout the performance of this exercise.
- Avoid throwing the dumbbell by using your legs or swinging your torso. Movement should only occur around your wrist joint.

WRIST EXTENSION

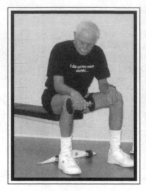 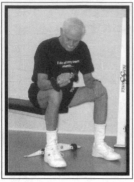

Start/Finish Position   Mid-Range Position

Muscles Influenced: wrist extensors

Suggested Repetitions: 8 - 12

Start/Finish Position: Grasp a dumbbell with your right hand. Sit down near the end of a bench (or a chair or stool) and place the front of your right forearm directly over your right upper leg so that your palm is facing down. Position your right wrist over your right kneecap. Lean forward slightly so that the angle between your upper and lower arms is about 90 degrees or less.

Performance Description: Pull the dumbbell up as high as possible by bending your wrist. Pause briefly in this mid-range position (your hand up) and then lower the dumbbell under control to the start/finish position (your hand down). After performing a set with your right arm, repeat the exercise for the other side of your body.

Training Tips:

• Keep your forearm directly over your upper leg throughout the performance of this exercise.

• Avoid throwing the dumbbell by using your leg or swinging your torso. Movement should only occur around your wrist joint.

FINGER FLEXION

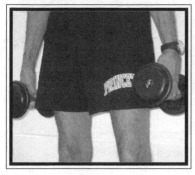
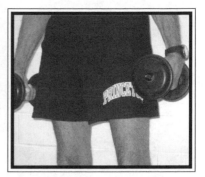

Start/Finish Position   Mid-Range Position

Muscles Influenced: finger flexors

Suggested Repetitions: 8 - 12

Start/Finish Position: Grasp a dumbbell with each hand. Hold the dumbbells near the sides of your upper legs with your palms facing each other. Spread your feet about shoulder-width apart. Straighten your arms and allow the dumbbells to roll down your hands to your fingertips.

Performance Description: Keeping your arms fairly straight, pull the dumbbells up to your thumbs. Pause briefly in this mid-range position (your fingers bent) and then lower the dumbbells under control to the start/finish position (your fingers straight).

Training Tips:

- Avoid throwing the dumbbells by using your legs or arms. Movement should only occur around your finger joints.

- Squeeze the dumbbells as hard as possible in the mid-range position.

- Lower the dumbbells all the way down to your fingertips.

- Do this exercise with one limb at a time if you have an arm injury, a gross difference in the strength between your limbs or desire a training variation.

PINCH GRIP

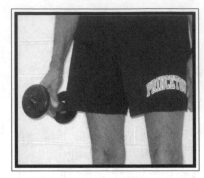

Start/Finish Position

Muscles Influenced: finger flexors

Suggested Time: 50 - 70 seconds

Start/Finish Position: Grasp the handle of a dumbbell with the fingertips and thumb of your right hand. Hold the dumbbell near the side of your upper leg with your palm facing your leg. Spread your feet about shoulder-width apart and straighten your right arm.

Performance Description: Remain in the start/finish position for the suggested amount of time. After performing a set with your right hand, repeat the exercise for the other side of your body.

Training Tips:

- Squeeze the dumbbell as hard as possible.

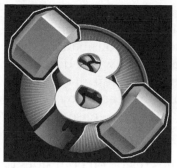

MODIFY YOUR MID-SECTION

The muscles of the abdominals and lower back serve as an important link between your lower body and torso. Collectively, these muscles form what has become known as your "core."

MUSCLES OF THE ABDOMINALS

The abdominal muscles are located on the anterior portion of your mid-section and are comprised of the rectus abdominis, obliques and transversus abdominis. These muscles perform a variety of functions.

Rectus Abdominis

This long, narrow muscle extends vertically across the front of your abdomen from the lower rim of your rib cage to your pelvis. Its

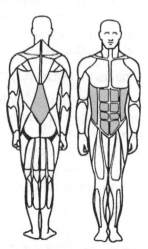

main function is torso flexion (pulling your torso toward your lower body). The fibers of this muscle are interrupted along their course by three horizontal fibrous bands which gives rise to the term "washboard abs" when describing an especially well-developed abdomen. The rectus abdominis helps to control your breathing and plays a major role in forced expiration during intense exercise.

Obliques

The external and internal obliques reside on both sides of your mid-section. The external oblique is a broad muscle; its fibers form a V across the front of your abdominal area, extending diagonally downward from your lower ribs to your pubic bone. The external oblique has two main functions: torso lateral flexion (bending your torso to the same side) and torso rotation (turning your torso to the opposite side). The internal oblique is located immediately under the external oblique on both sides of your abdomen; its fibers form an inverted V along the front of your abdominal wall, extending diagonally upward from your pubic bone to your ribs. The internal oblique has two main functions: torso lateral flexion (bending your torso to the same side) and torso rotation (turning your torso to the same side). In short, your external and internal obliques are used during movements in which your torso bends laterally or twists. These muscles are also active during expiration and inspiration, respectively.

Transversus Abdominis

The innermost layer of your abdominal musculature is the transversus abdominis. The fibers of this muscle run horizontally across your abdomen. The primary function of the transversus abdominis is to constrict your abdomen. This muscle is also involved in forced expiration and helps to control your breathing.

MUSCLES OF THE LOWER BACK

The lower back muscles are located on the posterior portion of your mid-section. Today, low-back pain remains one of the most common and costly medical problems. It has been estimated that 80% of the world's population will experience low-back pain sometime in their lives. Insufficient strength seems to be a factor related to low-back pain.

Erector Spinae

The main muscles in your lower back are the erector spinae (or "spinal erectors"). Their primary purpose is torso extension (straightening your torso from a bent-over position). However, the erector spinae also assist in torso lateral flexion (bending your torso to the same side) and torso rotation (turning your torso to the same side).

EXERCISES FOR THE MID-SECTION

This chapter will describe and illustrate four exercises that you can perform for the muscles of your mid-section. The exercises are the crunch, rotary crunch, side bend and stiff-leg deadlift.

CRUNCH

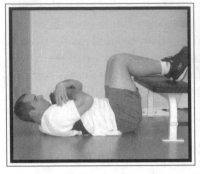 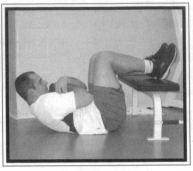

Start/Finish Position   *Mid-Range Position*

Muscles Influenced: rectus abdominis and iliopsoas

Suggested Repetitions: 10 - 12

Start/Finish Position: Grasp a dumbbell with both hands. Lie down on the floor and place the backs of your lower legs on the back pad of a bench (or a chair or stool). Position your upper legs so that they're approximately perpendicular to the floor and the angle between your upper and lower legs is about 90 degrees. Position the dumbbell on your chest and hold it in place. Bring your head toward your chest so that the upper portion of your shoulder blades doesn't touch the floor.

Performance Description: Pull your torso as close to your upper legs as possible. Pause briefly in this mid-range position (your torso near your upper legs) and then lower your torso under control to the start/finish position (your torso on the floor).

Training Tips:

- Avoid snapping your head forward as you perform this exercise. Movement should only occur around your hip joint and mid-section.
- Perform this exercise without the dumbbell if you cannot do 12 repetitions.
- Avoid this exercise if you have low-back pain.

ROTARY CRUNCH

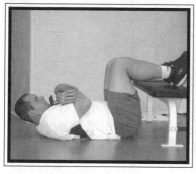
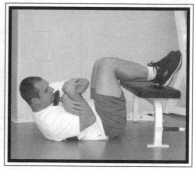

Start/Finish Position   *Mid-Range Position*

Muscles Involved: obliques and erector spinae (lower back)

Suggested Repetitions: 10 - 12

Start/Finish Position: Grasp a dumbbell with both hands. Lie down on the floor and place the backs of your lower legs on the back pad of a bench (or a chair or stool). Position your upper legs so that they're approximately perpendicular to the floor and the angle between your upper and lower legs is about 90 degrees. Position the dumbbell on your chest and hold it in place. Bring your head toward your chest so that the upper portion of your shoulder blades doesn't touch the floor.

Performance Description: Rotate your left shoulder as close to your right upper leg as possible. Pause briefly in this mid-range position (your torso rotated to the right) and then lower your torso under control to the start/finish position (your torso on the floor). After performing a set for the right side of your abdomen, repeat the exercise for the other side of your abdomen (rotating your torso to the left).

Training Tips:

- Perform this exercise without the dumbbell if you cannot do 12 repetitions.
- Avoid this exercise if you have low-back pain.

SIDE BEND

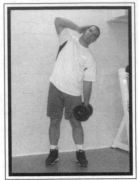 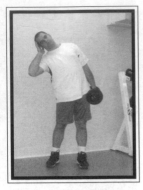

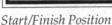

Start/Finish Position   *Mid-Range Position*

Muscles Influenced: obliques and erector spinae (lower back)

Suggested Repetitions: 10 - 12

Start/Finish Position: Grasp a dumbbell with your left hand. Hold the dumbbell against the side of your upper leg with your palm facing your leg. Spread your feet about shoulder-width apart and straighten your left arm. Place your right palm against the right side of your head. Without moving your hips, bend your torso to the left as far as possible.

Performance Description: Without moving your hips, bring your torso to the right as far as possible. Pause briefly in this mid-range position (your torso bent to the right) and then lower the dumbbell under control to the start/finish position (your torso bent to the left). After performing a set with the right side of your mid-section, repeat the exercise for the other side of your mid-section (holding the dumbbell in your right hand).

Training Tips:

- Avoid throwing the weight by moving your hips. Movement should only occur around your mid-section.
- Refrain from bending forward at the waist as you perform this exercise.
- Keep your feet flat on the floor as you perform this exercise.
- Avoid this exercise if you have low-back pain.

STIFF-LEG DEADLIFT

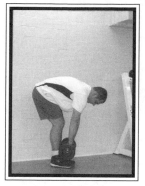 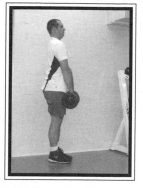

Start/Finish Position   *Mid-Range Position*

Muscles Influenced: erector spinae (lower back), gluteus maximus (buttocks) and hamstrings

Suggested Repetitions: 10 - 15

Start/Finish Position: Spread your feet slightly narrower than shoulder-width apart and point them straight ahead. Lower your torso and straighten your legs – but don't "lock" them. Grasp a dumbbell with each hand. Place most of your bodyweight on your heels. Straighten your arms and point your palms toward your legs.

Performance Description: Stand upright until your torso is almost completely straight. Pause briefly in this mid-range position (your torso almost completely straight) and then lower the dumbbells under control to the start/finish position (your torso bent).

Training Tips:

- Keep your arms and legs straight as you perform this exercise. Unlike the deadlift, your lower back should do most of the work.

- Exert force through your heels, not the balls of your feet.

- Use wrist straps if you have difficulty in maintaining your grip on the dumbbells.

- Avoid this exercise if you have low-back pain, hyperextended elbows or an exceptionally long torso and/or legs.

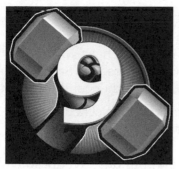

PUTTING IT ALL TOGETHER

Now that you understand the basics of improving your strength and fitness with dumbbells as well as learning many different exercises and their variants, you can learn the best ways of putting it all together. Let's take a look at some important considerations.

SCHEDULING WORKOUTS

There are several different ways to schedule your workouts based on your personal, professional and familial obligations. Sometimes, having set training days isn't always feasible. So, here are a few examples of how you can schedule your workouts to best meet your needs:

- *Two workouts per week:* You can do your workouts on any two non-consecutive days such as Monday/Thursday, Monday/Friday, Tuesday/Friday, Tuesday/Saturday or some other combination. If possible, try to spread out the two workouts so that the time between them is roughly the same. If your two workouts for the week come on Monday and Wednesday, for example, then you'll have to wait five days to work out again.

- *Three workouts per week*: You can do your workouts on any three non-consecutive days such as Monday/Wednesday/Friday, Monday/Wednesday/Saturday, Tuesday/Thursday/Sunday or some other combination.

- *One workout every third day*: With this schedule, simply think in terms of days between workouts rather than a specific day of the week to work out. You can do your workouts on Monday, Thursday, Sunday, Wednesday, Saturday, Tuesday, Friday and so on. In a three-week period, then, you'll get seven workouts: One week in which you do three workouts and two weeks in which you do two workouts.

- *One workout every 4 - 7 days*. Although this isn't an ideal scenario, it certainly beats doing nothing at all. Believe it or not, many people can use this type of infrequent training and still make significant improvements in their strength and fitness.

You should schedule your workouts for twice per week, every other day, every third day or whatever best fits your agenda. The idea is to make the best of the approach that allows you to individualize your program while providing your body with enough time to recover from your previ-

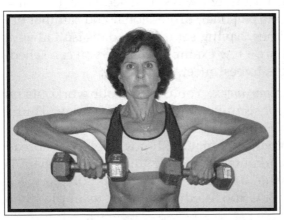

Figure 9.1: The amount of time that a muscle is exercised – or "loaded" – in a set is actually of greater importance than the number of repetitions that a muscle does.

ous workout so that you don't become overtrained. Remember, success comes from being consistent, working hard in each and every session and focusing on making progress. Not only will you improve your strength from this type of training but your level of fitness and overall health will increase dramatically as well.

Keep in mind that to this point, the discussions about scheduling are based on total-body workouts. Another option that's widely used is to do a split routine in which the body is "split" into different segments. Traditionally, split routines involve training different muscles on different days such as the chest on one day, the upper back on another and so on. For many individuals, this can be devastating since it doesn't allow for adequate recovery. Plus, more trips to the gym are required which can be a burden – especially for those who find it difficult enough to schedule workouts as it is. That said, some people might find that split routines are more favorable. Doing a total-body workout necessitates a focused effort that some individuals may find too exhausting to do in one day. Similarly, individuals who are engaged in sports or activities that place excessive demands on their hips and legs – such as biking and running – may be better off training their lower body once per week and their upper body twice per week to allow those muscles more time to recover. Also, splitting one total-body workout in two – preferably, a lower-body workout and an upper-body workout – may enable some people to focus on their weak points and/or include exercises that they were unable to do in a total-body workout. And, of course, some people simply opt to do a split routine as a matter of personal preference. A few words of caution however: Splitting up the body in this fashion isn't an open invitation to increase the volume of your training in terms of doing additional exercises/sets and workouts; rather, it's a means in which you can increase the diversity of your training.

TIME/REPETITIONS

With respect to doing a set of an exercise, people often ask, "How many repetitions?" But technically, they should ask, "How much time?" Yes, the amount of time that a muscle is exercised – or "loaded" – in a set is actually of greater importance than the number of repetitions that a muscle does. Think about it: Suppose that you and a friend both did 10 repetitions in the overhead press with 30-pound dumbbells. On the surface, it would seem as if both of you received the same degree of stimulation. But what if your 10 repetitions took 60 seconds to do and your friend's took 20 seconds? You both did the same number of repetitions and you both used the same weight but, obviously, you received more benefit from the exercise than your friend since your muscles were loaded for a longer period of time.

The time that a muscle is loaded has become known as "time under load" or "TUL." For the most part, it's not practical to do an exercise for a certain amount of time. (A notable exception would be performing an exercise that involves a "static hold" or isometric contraction such as the wall sit and pinch grip.) A more pragmatic way is to express the TUL as repetitions or a repetition range. So if a TUL of 60 seconds is desired and each repetition takes six seconds to perform, then some quick math reveals that the number of repetitions would be 10.

It's often suggested that the hips respond best to about 15 - 20 repetitions (or 90 - 120 seconds of TUL); the legs and lower back to about 10 - 15 repetitions (or 60 - 90 seconds of TUL); and the torso (the chest, upper back, shoulders and mid-section) to about 8 - 12 repetitions (or 50 - 70 seconds of TUL). Understand that these repetition ranges and TULs are merely recommendations that have been determined from the basic requirements of anaerobic activity (physical exertion that's characterized by brief but intense efforts such as strength training). Keep in mind, too, that there are exceptions to this based on individual needs. Note that the aforementioned repetition ranges are based on a six-second repetition: a two-second positive phase and a four-second negative phase (excluding, of course, the brief pause in the start/finish and mid-range positions).

These time frames allow for an inherent warm-up and a safe performance of the exercise while providing a significant stimulus to the targeted muscle. However, we're all individuals and vary somewhat in our response to strength training – both physically as well as mentally. As a result, you can – and should – utilize a

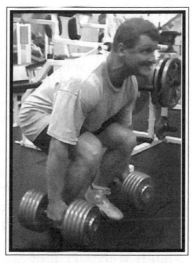

Figure 9.2: Placing progressively greater demands on your muscles is an absolute requirement for improving your strength.

variety of repetition ranges and TULs for optimum gains. Indeed, many individuals modify their repetition ranges based on their personal experiences and preferences along with a means of adding variety and new challenges to their training.

Some people prefer to use repetition ranges that are a bit higher than what's outlined here. Kim Wood, who was the Strength Coach of the Cincinnati Bengals from 1975-2003, has stated, "To maximally stimulate the lower body, it takes lots of repetitions – maybe a repetition range of 30 - 50 or more! Of course, this is very hard work . . . but everything you do should be 'all-out.'" And then, of course, some people prefer to use repetition ranges that are a bit lower than what's outlined here. The bottom line is that you can vary repetition ranges as long as the safety and efficacy of the exercise aren't compromised.

Many individuals opt for repetition speeds that are slower than a two-second positive and a four-second negative (a

2/4 speed) and count TULs rather than repetitions. If you choose to employ slower-speed repetitions in your program, you can use a mixture of cadences such as a 4/4 or an 8/8 speed. Other popular cadences include 5/5, 10/5, 10/10 and 4/4/4 speeds. (If three digits are given, the middle digit indicates the number of seconds to pause in the mid-range position.) Or, you can use whatever cadence that you prefer. Remember, there's no exact speed that has to be used. The only thing that really matters is that the speed of movement is safe and effective. In any event, if you choose a 10-second positive and a five-second negative for each repetition, then that's a total of 15 seconds per repetition (or a little more with brief pauses at the start/finish and mid-range positions). So in an exercise such as the deadlift with a TUL of about 90 - 120 seconds, a corresponding repetition range for a 10/5 speed would be about 6 - 8.

You're encouraged to experiment with varying the recommended repetition ranges and TULs along with implementing slower-speed repetitions. This will offer you new challenges in your quest for improved strength and fitness.

PROGRESSIVE DEMANDS

Placing progressively greater demands on your muscles is an absolute requirement for improving your strength. This tenet is put into practice by implementing the Double-Progressive Technique. The term "double progressive" refers to either increasing the resistance that you use or the repetitions that you do.

To illustrate this technique, suppose that your repetition range in the overhead press is 8 - 12. Also suppose that in today's workout, you did 12 repetitions to the point of muscular fatigue with 50-pound dumbbells in that exercise. Since you reached the upper limit of your repetition range, this means that you should increase the resistance for your next workout. Let's say that in your next workout, you get 11 repetitions to the point of muscular fatigue with 52.5-pound dumbbells. Since you didn't reach the upper limit of your repetition range, this means that you should keep the resistance the same for your next workout and try to do more than 11 repetitions. Thus, you have the double progression of either resistance or repetitions. To summarize: Whenever you can do the maximum number of repetitions in an exercise, increase the resistance for your next workout; whenever you cannot do the maximum number of repetitions in an exercise, keep the resistance the same for your next workout but try to do more repetitions.

Ideally, you should increase the resistance by about 5% whenever you reach your repetition goal. But what if you're unable to microload (as described in Chapter 1) and forced to increase the resistance more than the preferred 5%? If this is the case, it's recommended that you do at least 15 repetitions for upper-body exercises and 25 repetitions for lower-body exercises. This will make it safer when you progress in resistance. Here's an example of why: Recall the previous scenario in which your repetition range is 8 - 12 in the overhead press and you did 12 repetitions to the point of muscular fatigue with 50-pound dumbbells. But now, 52.5-pound dumbbells aren't available and you must use the 55-pounders. Going from 50-pound dumbbells to 55-pound dumbbells is a 10% increase and you may find

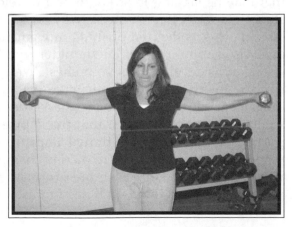

Figure 9.3: Single-joint movements should be used to pre-/post-exhaust a muscle.

yourself struggling with this resistance in an effort to get eight repetitions with good technique. It would be smarter and safer for you to implement a higher repetition range, waiting until you can perform 15 repetitions or more in the overhead press with the 50-pound dumbbells before progressing to the 55-pound dumbbells. At that point, your level of strength will be more capable of handling the heavier load. This tactic can serve well for many individuals, especially beginners who are learning how to work hard and handle progressively heavier weights.

INCORPORATING VARIETY

Staying enthusiastic about training is often a mental and physical challenge, especially when you do the "same old, same old." This suggests that variety is important in maintaining enthusiasm and overcoming plateaus.

As mentioned earlier, you can incorporate variety into your training by changing repetition ranges, TULs and repetition speeds. What follows are additional ways to vary your training.

Order of Exercise

Another option that works well is to periodically modify the order in which you perform your exercises. By switching the sequence, you can focus on exercises and body parts that may be lagging in strength and development. For instance, suppose that you've always done the supine (flat bench) press as the first pushing movement in your workout. Also suppose that your shoulders don't seem to be as strong or as developed as your chest. Well, you can prioritize the overhead press and make it your first pushing movement while the supine press becomes your secondary focus. This isn't to suggest that the supine press isn't important or imply that continued improvement in the supine press isn't a goal; you're merely changing the order of your exercises to emphasize the overhead press.

It must be noted that you'll need to use less weight in an

exercise when you do it later in your workout; similarly, you'll need to use more weight in an exercise when you do it earlier in your workout. So whenever you change the arrangement of exercises in your workout, you'll need to make appropriate adjustments in the weights that you use. Of course, your goal is to improve both movements in this new sequence. If you get to the point where you can use the same amount of weight for the same number of repetitions in an exercise when you do it later in a

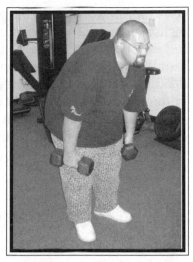

Figure 9.4: Periodically incorporating a workout theme will help you to round out your variety.

workout, then you've certainly gotten stronger. You can then take this newfound focus and stay with it for a few workouts, weeks or months or until you become stale or reach a plateau - which would be your cue to make changes again for continued progress.

Specialization Routines

An excellent means of stimulating growth and enjoying workouts is to "specialize." This allows you to hone in on your workouts and really concentrate on a muscle. You can prioritize your shoulders for a period of time, for example. Overall, you'd do the same volume of exercises in your workouts but with a greater emphasis on your shoulders. Understand that this doesn't exclude you from training the rest of your body nor does it require you to perform extra exercises or add more workouts.

As an added note, specialization routines aren't exclusive to focusing on a particular muscle. Individual exercises can be spotlighted and lend a zest to training. For instance, you may currently be using 50-pound dumbbells for 20 repetitions in the deadlift with a goal of 50-pound dumbbells for 30 repetitions. Then, you'd prioritize the deadlift and work towards your new goal by specializing in this lift until your goal is met.

Two sample specialization workouts – one for the shoulders and another for the arms – would look like this:

Shoulder Specialization Workout

Deadlift - 1 x 15
Decline Press - 1 x 12
Bent-Over Row - 1 x 12 (each arm)
Front Raise - 1 x 12
Upright Row - 1 x 12
Bent-Over Raise - 1 x 12 (each arm)
Shrug - 1 x 15
Side Bend - 1 x 15 (each side)
Wrist Flexion - 1 x 15 (each arm)
Wrist Extension - 1 x 15 (each arm)

Arm Specialization Workout

Squat - 1 x 25 (each leg)
Overhead Press - 1 x 10
Tricep Extension - 1 x 10 (each arm)
Supine Press - 1 x 10
Bench Row - 1 x 10
Bicep Curl - 1 x 10
Hammer Curl - 1 x 10
Side Bend - 1 x 12 (each side)

Performance Points:

• Do the overhead press, tricep extension and supine press with as little recovery as possible between the exercises; do the bench row, bicep curl and hammer curl with as little recovery as possible between the exercises.

The Pre-Exhaust Technique

Essentially, there are two types of exercise movements: primary and compound. A single-joint (or primary) movement involves a range of motion around only one joint; a multiple-joint (or compound) movement involves ranges of motion around more than one joint. The Pre-Exhaust Technique – which was first popularized in the early 1970s – employs what has been called a "double set": one single-joint movement coupled with a multiple-joint movement. The idea is to "pre-exhaust" a muscle by doing a single-joint movement followed quickly by a multiple-joint movement. For instance, you'd do a set of the shrug to pre-fatigue your trapezius and then immediately do a set of the upright row. Other "double sets" that incorporate the Pre-Exhaust Technique include any bent-arm fly coupled with an allied press for the chest (in other words, an incline fly would be followed by an incline press), the pullover coupled with the bent-over row and the wrist extension coupled with the reverse curl.

Here's a sample workout that utilizes the Pre-Exhaust Technique for the hips/legs, chest, upper back, shoulders and abdominals:

Pre-Exhaust Workout

Ball Squat - 1 x 20
Deadlift - 1 x 20
Supine Fly - 1 x 15
Supine Press - 1 x 10
Pullover - 1 x 15
Bent-Over Row - 1 x 10 (each arm)
Front Raise - 1 x 15
Overhead Press - 1 x 10
Standing Calf Raise - 1 x 15 (each leg)
Side Bend - 1 x 15 (each side)
Crunch - 1 x 20

Performance Points:

- Do these exercises with as little recovery as possible between the two: the ball squat and deadlift; the supine fly and supine press; the pullover and bent-over row; the front raise and overhead press; and the side bend and crunch.

The Post-Exhaust Technique

The opposite of the Pre-Exhaust Technique is the Post-Exhaust Technique. Here, the idea is to "post-exhaust" a muscle by doing a multiple-joint movement followed quickly by a single-joint movement. "Double sets" that incorporate the Post-Exhaust Technique include any press for the chest coupled with an allied bent-arm fly (in other words, a supine press would be followed by a supine fly), the overhead press coupled with the lateral raise and the bench row coupled with the pullover.

Here's a sample workout that utilizes the Post-Exhaust Technique for the hips/legs, chest, upper back, shoulders and abdominals:

Post-Exhaust Workout

Squat - 1 x 25 (each leg)
Stiff-Leg Deadlift - 1 x 25
Incline Press - 1 x 10
Incline Fly - 1 x 15
Bench Row - 1 x 10
Pullover - 1 x 15
Overhead Press - 1 x 10
Lateral Raise - 1 x 15
Seated Calf Raise - 1 x 15 (each leg)
Crunch - 1 x 15
Side Bend - 1 x 15 (each side)

Performance Points:

- Do these exercises with as little recovery as possible between the two: the squat and stiff-leg deadlift; the incline press and incline fly; the bench row and pullover;

the overhead press and lateral raise; and the crunch and side bend.

The Rest-Pause Technique

Another method that can be used to vary your training is the Rest-Pause Technique. Here's how: Pick a weight that will allow you to do a certain number of repetitions such as 12. After performing a set to fatigue and achieving your 12-repetition goal, take two or three deep breaths (about 10 seconds) and then attempt to do as many repetitions as possible. A key to remember is to keep your hands on the dumbbells. You can put the dumbbells down but keep them in your grasp so that you can stay focused on your breathing and the task ahead. Most people will be able to get a few more repetitions with this brief respite. If you're feeling up to it, take another short rest and then get as many repetitions as possible. If you focus on achieving a total of 20 repetitions with this weight, you'll be amazed at what your mind can do to make you achieve your goal. Don't be fooled by the simplicity of this technique: It's terribly difficult to do and will engrave the concept of "hard work" on the cornerstone of your training.

Workout Themes

Periodically incorporating a workout theme will help you to round out your variety. Themes can range from something such as a "50s Day" where you do 50 consecutive repetitions in all of your exercises to a "Grip Day" where you really emphasize working your gripping muscles (those that affect your wrists, hands and fingers). Sample 50s and grip workouts would look like this:

50s Workout

Ball Squat - 1 x 50
Incline Press - 1 x 50
Pullover - 1 x 50
Shrug - 1 x 50

Hammer Curl - 1 x 50
Seated Calf Raise - 1 x 50 (each leg)
Crunch - 1 x 50

Grip Workout

Overhead Press - 1 x 15 (each arm)
Bent-Over Row - 1 x 15 (each arm)
Supine Press - 1 x 10
Shrug - 1 x 20
Reverse Curl - 1 x 20
Wrist Flexion - 1 x 20 (each arm)
Deadlift - 1 x 30
Finger Flexion - 1 x 20
Crunch - 1 x 15

FINAL NOTES

As mentioned previously, having variety in your workouts is a great way to keep progressing and maintain a high level of enthusiasm. It's a good idea to have different workouts from which to choose and focus on over the course of time. For example, you can design three workouts and use a different one on each of your three training days. You can implement specialization programs, themes or other training techniques whenever you want as long as your programs are well rounded and your workouts are progressively more challenging.

Remember, your workouts should be something that suit your individual tastes and are enjoyable. If you don't find that an exercise is mentally stimulating, there's no reason that you "have to" perform it just because it's recommended. Yes, some exercises are more demanding than others and, for that very reason, are extremely productive. But if you're not going to focus when you perform that exercise, you'll risk injuring yourself and your progress will be slow at best. Make it a point to have a well-rounded approach to your training to achieve good joint stability, flexibility, strength and enjoyment. Make your training meaningful; train with a purpose.

The importance of progression suggests that that you should keep track of your efforts. You can use something as simple as a spiral notebook to record your exercises, performance (specifically, the resistance and repetitions), bodyweight and workout duration as well as any additional comments. Keeping this log will provide you with feedback and motivation which will enable you to analyze your program and its effectiveness. If you're making progress, it will be reflected in your log and you'll know that your program is working. On the other hand, the information in your log can reveal that something is amiss and corrective measures must be taken. Here's an example: If your records indicate that you're able to do 20 repetitions in the stiff-leg deadlift, you should strive to increase the resistance, repetitions or both for the next workout or two. If over the course of several workouts your progress has stalled or you're starting to regress, you may need to alter your program in some way. Or, it may be a sign that you need to take a few additional days of recovery. This information will allow you to tweak your program in an intelligent manner and make any necessary adjustments.

Speaking of recovery, many of the preceding techniques are very demanding on your body and recovery ability. So while the techniques are a valuable means of improving your strength and fitness, you should use them intelligently and sparingly.

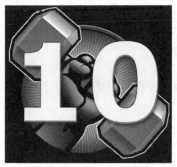

WORKOUTS FOR THE TOTAL BODY

This chapter shares an extensive array of total-body workouts with dumbbells that were contributed by strength and fitness professionals from across the United States. While their "recipes" are different, all of the workouts maintain the same fundamental qualities of a safe, effective and efficient approach to improving strength and fitness. Follow the guidelines that are expressed throughout this book and experiment with as many of the workouts as possible to determine what best suits your individual tastes and needs.

Many of the contributors have included brief points concerning how the workouts are to be performed. Unless otherwise specified, all workouts are based on taking each set to the point of muscular fatigue. In addition, you should perform each repetition in a deliberate, controlled manner. If a specific speed of movement is recommended, it's usually designated by two numbers such as 2/4. The first digit refers to the number of seconds that it should take to raise the weight and the last digit refers to the number of seconds that it should take to lower the weight. (If three digits are given, the middle digit indicates the number of seconds to pause in the mid-range position.)

Total-Body Workout #1 (Steve Baldwin)

Ball Squat - 1 x 20
Lunge - 1 x 20 (each leg)
Standing Calf Raise - 1 x 20 (each leg)
Overhead Press - 1 x 12-15
Bent-Over Row - 1 x 12-15 (each arm)
Supine Press - 1 x 12-15
Shrug - 1 x 20
Bicep Curl - 1 x 12-15
Bent-Over Raise - 1 x 12-15 (each arm)
External Rotation - 1 x 20 (each arm)
Stiff-Leg Deadlift - 1 x 20
Crunch - 1 x 20
Wrist Flexion - 1 x 20 (each arm)
Wrist Extension - 1 x 20 (each arm)

Performance Points:

- Use a 3/3 speed for all of the exercises.

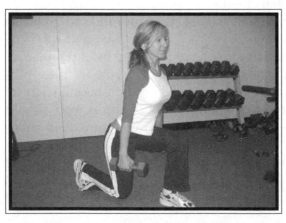

Figure 10.1: It's often suggested that the hips respond best to about 15-20 repetitions (or 90-120 seconds of TUL).

Total-Body Workout #2 (Drew Baye)

Deadlift - 1 x 8-12
Stiff-Leg Deadlift - 1 x 8-12
Standing Calf Raise - 1 x 8-12 (each leg)
Bent-Over Row - 1 x 5-8 (each arm)
Overhead Press - 1 x 5-8
Shrug - 1 x 5-8
Supine Press - 1 x 5-8
Bicep Curl - 1 x 5-8
French Curl - 1 x 5-8 (each arm)
Wrist Flexion - 1 x 5-8 (each arm)
Wrist Extension - 1 x 5-8 (each arm)
Crunch - 1 x 8-12

Performance Points:

- Use a 2/4 speed for all of the exercises.

Total-Body Workout #3 (Randy Berning)

Squat - 1 x 20 (each leg)
Bent-Over Row - 1 x 10 (each arm)
Supine Bench - 1 x 10
Front Raise - 1 x 10
Shrug - 1 x 10
Lateral Raise - 1 x 10
Hammer Curl - 1 x 10
Lunge - 1 x 10 (each leg)
Squat - 1 x 20 (each leg)

Performance Points:

- On the first set of the squat, do 20 repetitions but stop before you reach the point of muscular fatigue. On the second set of the squat, use the most weight that you can lift for 10 repetitions and go to muscular fatigue. Take about 30 seconds of recovery. Use the same weight and go to muscular fatigue. Continue to do the exercise in this fashion until you achieve a total of 20 repetitions.

Total-Body Workout #4 (Randy Berning)

Upright Row - 1 x 10
Overhead Press - 1 x 10 (alternating style)
Bicep Curl - 1 x 10
Pullover - 1 x 10
Bent-Over Raise - 1 x 10 (each arm)
Deadlift - 1 x 20
Overhead Press - 1 x 10 (alternating style)
Bicep Curl - 1 x 10
Pullover - 1 x 10
Bent-Over Raise - 1 x 10 (each arm)
Deadlift - 1 x 20

Performance Points:

- On the first set of the deadlift, do 20 repetitions but stop before you reach the point of muscular fatigue. On the second set of the deadlift, use the most weight that you can lift for 10 repetitions and go to muscular fatigue. Take about 30 seconds of recovery. Use the same weight and go to muscular fatigue. Continue to do the exercise in this fashion until you achieve a total of 20 repetitions.

Total-Body Workout #5 (Randy Berning)

Lunge - 1 x 20 (each leg)
Shrug - 1 x 10
Incline Press - 1 x 10
Bent-Over Row - 1 x 10 (each arm)
Lateral Raise - 1 x 10
Hammer Curl - 1 x 10
Tricep Extension - 1 x 10 (each arm)
Lunge - 1 x 20 (each leg)

Performance Points:

- On the first set of the lunge, do 20 repetitions (with each leg) but stop before you reach the point of muscular fatigue. On the second set of the lunge, use the most weight

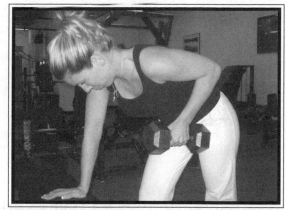

Figure 10.2: A major advantage of using dumbells is that it forces each of your limbs to work independently of the other.

that you can lift for 10 repetitions and go to muscular fatigue. Take about 30 seconds of recovery. Use the same weight and go to muscular fatigue. Continue to do the exercise in this fashion until you achieve a total of 20 repetitions (with each leg).

Total-Body Workout #6 (Michael Bradley)

Deadlift - 1 x 15
Lateral Raise - 1 x 10
Bent-Over Raise - 1 x 10 (each arm)
Front Raise - 1 x 10
Overhead Press - 1 x 8
Bent-Over Row - 1 x 8 (each arm)
Incline Press - 1 x 8
Shrug - 1 x 8
Crunch - 1 x 8

Total-Body Workout #7 (Brian Canaster)

Front Raise - 1 x 12-15
Incline Press - 2 x 8-12
Shrug - 1 x 12-15
Upright Row - 2 x 8-12
Lateral Raise – 1 x 12-15

Overhead Press - 2 x 8-12
Bicep Curl - 1 x 12-15
Bench Row - 2 x 8-12
Squat - 2 x 12-20 (each leg)
Lunge - 1 x 12-15 (each leg)
Deadlift - 2 x 12-20

Performance Points:

- Take about 20 - 30 seconds of recovery between each exercise.

Total-Body Workout #8 (Luke Carlson)

Deadlift - 1 x 20
Lunge - 1 x 8 (each leg)
Lateral Raise - 1 x 4-7
Overhead Press - 1 x 3-5
Bent-Over Row - 1 x 12 (each arm)
Supine Fly - 1 x 12
Supine Press - 1 x 6-8
Bicep Curl - 1 x 12 (alternating style)

Performance Points:

- Use a 5/5/5 speed for the lateral raise, a 10/10 speed for the overhead press, a 2/10 speed for the supine press and a 2/4 speed for all of the other exercises.

Total-Body Workout #9 (Michael De Joseph)

Deadlift - 1 x 12, 1 x 10, 1 x 8
Incline Press - 1 x 12, 1 x 10, 1 x 8
Pullover - 1 x 12, 1 x 10, 1 x 8
Lateral Raise - 1 x 12, 1 x 10, 1 x 8
Bicep Curl - 1 x 12, 1 x 10, 1 x 8

Performance Points:

- Increase the weight of the dumbbells for each set of an exercise (thus, the nickname of this workout is "Run the Rack").

- Take little or no recovery between sets and exercises. This will increase your level of intensity.

- The two keys of this workout are to use as much resistance as possible for the prescribed number of repetitions and to go to the point of muscular fatigue.

Total-Body Workout #10 (Jason Hadeed)

Upright Row to Overhead Press - 1 x 12-15 (each arm)
Bench Row - 1 x 12-15
Supine Press - 1 x 12-15
Bent-Over Raise - 2 x 12-15 (each arm)
Lateral Raise - 1 x 12-15
Front Raise - 1 x 12-15
Bicep Curl - 1 x 12-15
Tricep Extension - 1 x 12-15 (each arm)
Supine Press - 1 x 12-15
Lunge - 2 x 15-20 (each leg)
Stiff-Leg Deadlift - 2 x 15-20
Step-Up - 2 x 15-20 (each leg)
Lunge - 2 x 15-20 (each leg)
Standing Calf Raise - 2 x 50 (each leg)
Crunch - 1 x as many reps as possible

Performance Points:

- With your right arm, do one repetition of the upright row followed by one repetition of the overhead press (while standing). Then, do the same thing with your left arm. Continue this sequence until you perform 12 - 15 repetitions with each arm.

- In the bicep curl, raise the dumbbells with your palms facing upward. In the mid-range position, turn your hands and lower the dumbbells with your palms facing downward. Immediately after completing the tricep extension, do the supine press with the same weight.

Total-Body Workout #11 (Chip Harrison)

Deadlift - 1 x 15-20
Standing Calf Raise - 1 x 10-15 (each leg)
Supine Press - 1 x 8-12
Bent-Over Row - 1 x 8-12 (each arm)
Incline Press - 1 x 8-10
Bench Row - 1 x 8-10
Shrug - 1 x 10-12
Upright Row - 1 x 8-12
Tricep Extension - 1 x 8-12 (each arm)
Concentration Curl - 1 x 8-12 (each arm)
Wrist Extension - 1 x 10-12 (each arm)
Crunch - 1 x 8-12

TOTAL-BODY WORKOUT #12 (Aaron Hillman)

Shrug - 3 x 15
Incline Press - 3 x 10
Bent-Over Row - 3 x 10 (each arm)
Front Raise - 1 x 10
Lateral Raise - 1 x 10
Preacher Curl - 1 x 10 (each arm)
Tricep Extension - 1 x 10 (each arm)
Pinch Grip - 1 x 1 minute (each hand)
Squat - 2 x 12 (each leg)
Stiff-Leg Deadlift - 2 x 12
Standing Calf Raise - 2 x 15 (each leg)
Deadlift - 1 x 30

Performance Points:

- On the first set of the shrug, use the most weight that you can lift for 15 repetitions and go to the point of muscular fatigue. Repeat this for two more sets using lighter dumbbells while taking as little recovery as possible between the sets.

- Do the first set of the incline press with the bench at about a 60-degree angle. For the next two sets of that

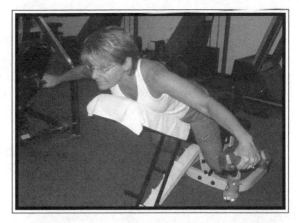

Figure 10.3:
Dumbbells and an
adjustable bench
give you numerous
options for training.

exercise, lower the angle of the bench so that the second set is done at about a 45-degree angle and the third set is done at about a 30-degree angle. Use the same weight for all three sets of this exercise while taking as little recovery as possible between the sets.

- In the bent-over row, take as little recovery as possible between the three sets. During the first three repetitions of the third set, hold the dumbbell in the mid-range position for 10 seconds.

- After the first three exercises, take about one minute of recovery between each set.

Total-Body Workout #13 (Gregg Humphreys)

Squat - 1 x 15 (each leg)
Deadlift - 1 x 10
Stiff-Leg Deadlift - 1 x 10
Bent-Over Row - 1 x 10 (each arm)
Incline Press - 1 x 10
Lateral Raise - 1 x 10
Bench Row - 1 x 10
Tricep Extension - 1 x 10 (each arm)
Bicep Curl - 4 x 10
Side Bend - 1 x 15 (each side)

Performance Points:

- On the first set of the bicep curl, use the most weight that you can lift for 10 repetitions and go to the point of muscular fatigue. Repeat this for three more sets using lighter dumbbells while taking as little recovery as possible between the sets.

TOTAL-BODY WORKOUT #14 (Tom Kelso)

Stiff-Leg Deadlift - 1 x 10-15
Deadlift - 1 x 15-20, 1 x 10-15
Supine Press - 1 x 8-14
Lateral Raise - 1 x 8-14
Bent-Over Row - 1 x 8-14 (each arm)
Overhead Press - 1 x 8-14 (alternating style)
Incline Press - 1 x 8-14
French Curl - 1 x 8-14 (each arm)
Bicep Curl - 1 x 8-14
Crunch - 1 x 15-20, 1 x 10-15

TOTAL-BODY WORKOUT #15 (Tom Kelso)

Supine Press - 1 x 10-15
Bench Row - 1 x 10-15
Overhead Press - 1 x 6-12
Bent-Over Row - 1 x 6-12 (each arm)
Incline Press - 1 x 6-12
Upright Row - 1 x 10-15
Squat - 1 x 10-15, 1 x 8-12 (each leg)
Standing Calf Raise - 1 x 15-20 (each leg)
Crunch - 1 x 20-25

Performance Points:

- You can alternate this workout with Total-Body Workout #14.

TOTAL-BODY WORKOUT #16 (Paul Kennedy)

Bent-Arm Fly - 1 x 8-12
Supine Press - 1 x 8-12
Pullover - 1 x 8-12
Bent-Over Row - 1 x 8-12 (each arm)
Lateral Raise - 1 x 8-12
Overhead Press - 1 x 8-12
Bicep Curl - 1 x 8-12
Tricep Kickback - 1 x 8-12 (each arm)
Squat - 1 x 10-15 (each leg)
Standing Calf Raise - 1 x 10-15 (each leg)
Deadlift - 1 x 10-15

Performance Points:

- The bent-arm fly, pullover, lateral raise, squat, standing calf raise and deadlift are required exercises in this workout.

- Instead of the supine press, you can also do the incline press or decline press. Instead of the bent-over row, you can also do the bench row. Instead of the overhead press, you can also do the upright row or front raise.

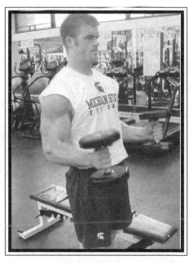

- Instead of the bicep curl, you can also do the concentration curl. Instead of the tricep kickback, you can also do the tricep extension.

- Instead of the squat, you can also do the ball squat. Instead of the deadlift, you can also do the step-up or lunge.

Figure 10.4: It's much safer and more effective to perform higher repetitions than it is to "max out."

- If you prefer, you can do up to three sets of each exercise by using the Quick Set System. This technique allows you to do a higher volume of training in a shorter period of time. In brief, the Quick Set System works like this: Go to the point of muscular fatigue on the first set and then reduce the resistance by about 25-30%. Do a second set – your first "quick set – with this lightened load to the point of muscular fatigue and then reduce the resistance by about 25-30%. Do a third set – your second "quick set" – with this lightened load to the point of muscular fatigue.

- So that there's no misunderstanding, the word "quick" describes how you should move between sets/exercises, not how you should do your repetitions. You should transition quickly from one set/exercise to the next but perform each repetition in a deliberate, controlled manner.

Total-Body Workout #17 (Sam Knopik)
Shrug - 1 x 8-12
Squat - 1 x 15-20 (each leg)
Standing Calf Raise - 1 x 15-20 (each leg)
Supine Press - 1 x 8-12
Bent-Over Row - 1 x 8-12 (each arm)
Overhead Press - 1 x 8-12
French Curl - 1 x 8-12 (each arm)
Bicep Curl - 1 x 8-12

Performance Points:

- If you stop a set before you reach the point of muscular fatigue, do a second set of the exercise.

Total-Body Workout #18 (Aaron Komarek)
Deadlift - 1 x 15-20
Stiff-Leg Deadlift - 1 x 15-20
Standing Calf Raise - 1 x 15-20 (each leg)

Supine Press - 1 x 10-15
Bent-Over Row - 1 x 10-15 (each arm)
Incline Press - 1 x 10-15
Pullover - 1 x 10-15
Overhead Press - 1 x 10-15
Bent-Over Raise - 1 x 10-15 (each arm)
External Rotation - 1 x 10-15 (each arm)
Wrist Extension - 1 x 10-15 (each arm)
Crunch - 1 x 15-20

Total-Body Workout #19 (Kristopher R. Kotch)

Deadlift - 1 x 15-20
Shrug - 1 x 8-12
Seated Calf Raise - 1 x 15-20 (each leg)
Upright Row - 1 x 8-12
Overhead Press - 1 x 8-12
Bent-Over Row - 1 x 8-12 (each arm)
Supine Fly - 1 x 8-12
Supine Press - 1 x 8-12
Bicep Curl - 1 x 8 12
French Curl - 1 x 8-12 (each arm)

Performance Points:

• If you prefer, you can do two sets of each exercise.

Total-Body Workout #20 (Mike Lawrence)

Supine Press - 1 x 8, 1 x 6
Bent-Over Raise - 1 x 12 (each arm)
Bench Row - 1 x 10
Incline Press - 1 x 8, 1 x 6
Bent-Over Raise - 1 x 12 (each arm)
Bench Row - 1 x 10
Overhead Press - 1 x 8, 1 x 6
Ball Squat - 1 x 12
Stiff-Leg Deadlift - 1 x 12
Ball Squat - 1 x 12

Stiff-Leg Deadlift - 1 x 12
Ball Squat - 1 x 12

Performance Points:

- Take as little recovery as possible between the bent-over raise and bench row. Take about 90 seconds of recovery between all of the other sets and exercises for the upper body.

- Take as little recovery as possible between the five exercises for the lower body.

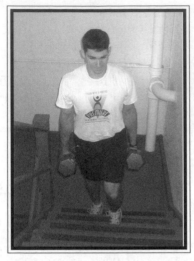

Figure 10.5: Athletes who become stronger will increase their potential to become better.

- As a variation, you can perform the ball squat with a speed of movement that's slower than usual (such as a 10/10 speed).

- You should be able to complete this workout in about 30 minutes or less.

- Insert your favorite mid-section exercises as a finisher for a well-balanced program that addresses the major muscular structures of your upper and lower bodies.

Total-Body Workout #21 (Ken Leistner)

Overhead Press - 1 x 12
Stiff-Leg Deadlift - 1 x 15
Bench Row - 1 x 12
Pullover - 1 x 15
Deadlift - 1 x 15
Upright Row - 1 x 12
Incline Press - 1 x 10
Bicep Curl - 1 x 12
Deadlift - 1 x 20

Total-Body Workout #22 (John Mikula)

Squat - 1 x 12-14 (each leg)
Lunge - 1 x 20-30 (each leg)
Dorsi Flexion - 1 x 12-14
Supine Press - 1 x 8-10
Bent-Over Row - 1 x 8-10 (each arm)
Overhead Press - 1 x 8-10
Lateral Raise - 1 x 10-12
Bent-Over Raise - 1 x 10-12 (each arm)
Shrug - 1 x 10-12
Front Raise - 1 x 12-14
Stiff-Leg Deadlift - 1 x 12-14

Performance Points:

- Take no more than about 30 - 90 seconds of recovery between each exercise.

- You should be able to complete this workout in about 45 minutes or less.

Total-Body Workout #23 (Willis Paine)

Lunge - 1 x 20-30 (each leg)
Standing Calf Raise - 1 x 20-30 (each leg)
Supine Press - 1 x 8-12
Bent-over Row - 1 x 8-12 (each arm)
Incline Press - 1 x 8-12
Bent-Over Raise - 1 x 8-12 (each arm)
Lateral Raise - 1 x 8-12
French Curl - 1 x 8-12 (each arm)
Bicep Curl - 1 x 8-12
Crunch - 1 x 20-30

Performance Points:

- Take as little recovery as possible between each exercise.

- You should be able to complete this workout in about 30 minutes or less.

Total-Body Workout #24 (Jeff Roudebush)

Deadlift - 1 x 25
Lunge - 1 x 15 (each leg)
Stiff-Leg Deadlift - 1 x 15
Standing Calf Raise - 1 x 15 (each leg)
Supine Press - 1 x 10
Incline Press - 1 x 10
Overhead Press - 1 x 10
French Curl - 1 x 10 (each arm)
Deadlift - 1 x 15
Upright Row - 1 x 10
Bent-Over Row - 1 x 10 (each arm)
Bicep Curl - 1 x 10 (alternating style)

Total-Body Workout #25 (Mike Shibinski)

Squat - 1 x 20 (each leg)
Deadlift - 1 x 15
Supine Fly - 1 x 12
Supine Press - 1 x 12
Pullover - 1 x 12
Bent-Over Row - 1 x 12 (each arm)
Lateral Raise - 1 x 12
Overhead Press - 1 x 12
Upright Row - 1 x 12
Shrug - 1 x 12
Bicep Curl - 1 x 10
Tricep Extension - 1 x 10 (each arm)
Preacher Curl - 1 x 10 (each arm)
Tricep Kickback - 1 x 10 (each arm)

Total-Body Workout #26 (Rob Spector)

Deadlift - 1-2 x 12-15
Overhead Press - 1-2 x 6-8
Bent-Over Row - 1-2 x 6-8 (each arm)
Supine Press - 1-2 x 6-8
Standing Calf Raise - 1-2 x 10-12 (each leg)

Crunch - 1 x 10-12
Pullover - 1 x 20
Supine Fly - 1 x 10-12

Total-Body Workout #27 (Scott Swanson)
Overhead Press - 1 x 8-10
Upright Row - 1 x 8-10
Incline Press - 1 x 8-10
Upright Row - 1 x 8-10
Incline Press - 1 x 8-10
Bench Row - 1 x 8-10
Incline Press - 1 x 8-10
Bench Row - 1 x 8-10
Supine Press - 1 x 8-10
Bench Row - 1 x 8-10
Step-Up - 2 x 8-10 (each leg)
Stiff-Leg Deadlift - 1 x 8-10
Lunge - 1 x 30 (each leg)
Shrug - 2 x 8-10

Performance Points:

- This workout begins with exercises done in an upright position and progressively lowers the angle of the push/pull until the exercises are done in a supine position (thus, the nickname of this workout is "Down the Ladder").

- Do the first set of the incline press with the bench at about a 75-degree angle. For the next two sets of that exercise, lower the angle of the bench so that the second set is done at about a 45-degree angle and the third set is done at about a 15-degree angle. Use the same protocol for the three sets of the bench row.

Total-Body Workout #28 (Scott Swanson)
Shrug - 1 x 15
Squat - 2 x 10 (each leg)
Stiff-Leg Deadlift - 2 x 10

Deadlift - 1 x 12-15
Incline Press - 2 x 6
Bent-Over Raise - 1 x 8 (each arm)
Supine Press - 1 x 8
Bent-Over Row - 1 x 8 (each arm)
Supine Press - 1 x 8
Bent-Over Row - 1 x 8 (each arm)
Lateral Raise - 1 x 10
Tricep Extension - 2 x 6 (each arm)
Preacher Curl - 2 x 6 (each arm)

Performance Points:

- This workout is a brutal, merciless attack on your muscular system (thus, the nickname of this workout is "Howitzer").

Total-Body Workout #29 (Scott Swanson)

Shrug - 1 x 12, 1 x 8, 1 x 4
Supine Bench - 1 x 10, 1 x 7, 1 x 4
Bent-Over Row - 1 x 10, 1 x 7, 1 x 4 (each arm)
Incline Press - 1 x 10, 1 x 7, 1 x 4
Pullover - 1 x 10, 1 x 7, 1 x 4
Overhead Press - 1 x 10, 1 x 7, 1 x 4
Bent-Over Raise - 1 x 10, 1 x 7 (each arm)
Hammer Curl to Overhead Press - 1 x 10
Squat - 1 x 10, 1 x 7, 1 x 4 (each leg)
Stiff-Leg Deadlift - 1 x 12, 1 x 10
Deadlift - 1 x 15
Stiff-Leg Deadlift - 1 x 8

Performance Points:

- This workout will strengthen and protect the vulnerable joints in your body (thus, the nickname of this workout is "Full Metal Jacket").

- Do one repetition of the hammer curl followed by one repetition of the overhead press (while standing). Continue this sequence until you perform 10 repetitions.

- Take no more than about 60 seconds of recovery between sets.

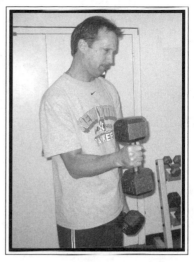

Figure 10.6: The object of a set is to stimulate as many muscle fibers as possible.

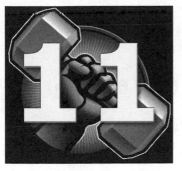

WORKOUTS WITH A TWIST

This chapter contains numerous workouts with dumb-bells that are based on the same safe, effective and efficient approach to improving strength and fitness that has been discussed throughout this book. As you'll see, however, these workouts involve a slight "twist." Included are work-outs that are designed to place exceptionally high demands on your musculoskeletal and cardiorespiratory systems as well as workouts for those who prefer to "split" their body parts or specialize in a body part or exercise. Follow the guidelines that are expressed throughout this book and experiment with as many of the workouts as possible to determine what best suits your individual tastes and needs.

Some of the workouts include brief points concerning how they're to be performed. Unless otherwise specified, all workouts are based on taking each set to the point of muscular fatigue. In addition, you should perform each repetition in a deliberate, controlled manner. If a specific speed of movement is recommended, it's usually designated by two numbers such as 2/4. The first digit refers to the number of seconds that it should take to raise the weight and the last digit refers to the number of seconds that it should take to lower the weight.

The One-Weight Workout (Fred Fornicola)

Overhead Press - 1 x 15
Stiff-Leg Deadlift
Bench Row
Supine Press
Shrug
Deadlift
Crunch

Performance Points:

• Use the same weight for all of the exercises (thus, the nickname of this workout is "One-Weight Workout"). The weight that you use should be one that you can do for at least 15 repetitions in the overhead press (while standing). Your levels of strength and conditioning will dictate the number of repetitions that you do in the subsequent exercises. For this reason, no specific target repetitions are listed. Needless to say, this workout can be extremely challenging to the ego.

• Try to keep your hands on the dumbbells for the entire workout.

• Take as little recovery as possible between each exercise.

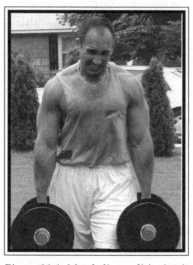

Figure 11.1: Metabolic conditioning is the ability to involve the musculoskeletal and cardiorespiratory systems simultaneously with intense workloads for a prescribed period of time.

- This workout is especially hard on your grip and overall musculature as well as your cardiorespiratory system.

3x3 Workout #1 (Matt Brzycki)

Deadlift - 1 x 20
Supine Press - 1 x 12
Bench Row - 1 x 12
Deadlift - 1 x 15
Supine Press - 1 x 10
Bench Row - 1 x 10
Deadlift - 1 x 12
Supine Press - 1 x 8
Bench Row - 1 x 8

Performance Points:

- This workout is a series of three exercises that are done a total of three times (thus, the nickname of this workout is "3x3" – which is read as "three by three"). Essentially, it consists of a multiple-joint movement for the hips followed by a multiple-joint movement for the chest followed by a multiple-joint movement for the upper back and repeated two more times. These three types of movements address virtually every major muscle in your body including your hips, hamstrings, quadriceps, chest, upper back, shoulders, biceps, triceps and forearms.

- This workout is extremely time-efficient; most variations can be performed in about 20 minutes or less.

- Use a 2/4 speed for all of the exercises.

- Take as little recovery as possible between each exercise.

- Don't be fooled by the simplicity of this type of workout. Though it may not appear so, a 3x3 Workout – if done as outlined here – can be incredibly challenging and demanding.

3x3 Workout #2 (Matt Brzycki)
Deadlift - 1 x 8
Incline Press - 1 x 8
Bench Row - 1 x 8
Ball Squat - 1 x 6
Supine Press - 1 x 6
Bench Row - 1 x 6
Deadlift - 1 x 5
Decline Press - 1 x 5
Bench Row - 1 x 5

Performance Points:
• Use an 8/8 speed for the deadlift and a 4/4 speed for the other exercises.

• Take as little recovery as possible between each exercise.

3x3 Workout #3 (Ken Mannie)
Deadlift - 1 x 15
Lunge - 1 x 10 (each leg)
Stiff-Leg Deadlift - 1 x 10
Incline Press - 1 x 8-10
Bent-Over Row - 1 x 8-10 (each arm)
Overhead Press - 1 x 8-10
Front Raise - 1 x 8-10
Lateral Raise - 1 x 8-10
Hammer Curl to Overhead Press - 1 x 8-10

Performance Points:
• Do one repetition of the hammer curl followed by one repetition of the overhead press (while standing). Continue this sequence until you perform 8 - 10 repetitions.

• Take about 2 - 3 minutes of recovery after the three exercises for the hips and legs and again after the first three exercises for the torso. Otherwise, take about two minutes of recovery between each exercise.

- Reduce the amount of recovery between exercises as tolerated.

Upper-Body Workout #1 (Jeff Friday)

Bench Press - 1 x 8-12
Bench Row - 1 x 8-12
Incline Press - 1 x 8-12
Bench Row - 1 x 8-12
Incline Press - 1 x 8-12
Bench Row - 1 x 8-12
Incline Press - 1 x 8-12
Lateral Raise - 1 x 8-12
Front Raise - 1 x 8-12
Internal Rotation - 1 x 8-12 (each arm)
External Rotation - 1 x 8-12 (each arm)
Overhead Press - 1 x 8-12
Bicep Curl - 1 x 8-12
Tricep Extension - 1 x 8-12 (each arm)

Performance Points:

- Do the first set of the incline press with the bench at about a 30-degree angle. For the next two sets of that exercise, raise the angle of the bench so that the second set is done at about a 45-degree angle and the third set is done at about a 60-degree angle.

Upper-Body Workout #2 (Sunir Jossan)

Supine Press - 1 x 10
Pullover - 1 x 10
Incline Press - 1 x 8
Bent-Over Row - 1 x 10 (each arm)
Overhead Press - 1 x 10, 1 x 8
Bicep Curl - 1 x 12
French Curl - 1 x 12 (each arm)
Bicep Curl - 1 x 10
Crunch - 1 x 20

Upper/Lower Split Workout #1 (Brian Conatser)

Supine Bench - 1 x 8
Bench Row - 1 x 8
Overhead Press - 1 x 8
Pullover - 1 x 8
Incline Fly - 1 x 8
Upright Row - 1 x 8
Lateral Raise - 1 x 8
Bent-Over Raise - 1 x 8 (each arm)

Squat - 1 x 15-20 (each leg)
Deadlift - 1 x 15-20
Lunge - 1 x 12-15 (each leg)
Step-Up - 1 x 12-15 (each leg)
Standing Calf Raise - 1 x 50 (each leg)

Performance Points:

- The upper-body and lower-body workouts are meant to be done on two separate days.

- Use a 2/8 speed for all of the eight exercises in the upper-body workout (thus, the nickname of this workout is "V-8").

- The lower-body workout of this split routine is extremely demanding (thus, the nickname of this workout is "Leg Lobotomy").

- Take about 20 - 30 seconds of recovery between each exercise.

Upper/Lower Split Workout #2 (Adam Rankin)

Shrug - 1 x 15, 1 x 10
Lateral Raise - 1 x 10
Front Raise - 1 x 10
Overhead Press - 1 x 10
Bent-Over Row - 1 x 10 (each arm)
Supine Press - 1 x 10
Bicep Curl - 1 x 10

Pullover – 1 x 15
Pinch Grip - 1 x 2 minutes (each hand)
Deadlift - 1 x 20

Lunge - 1 x 12 (each leg)
Wall Sit - 1 x 2 minutes
Step-Up - 1 x 12 (each leg)
Lunge - 1 x 12 (each leg)
Deadlift - 1 x 10

Performance Points:

- The upper-body and lower-body workouts are meant to be done on two separate days.

- Do all of the exercises to the point of muscular fatigue except for the first set of the shrug, the two sets of the lunge and the step-up.

Chest Specialization Workout (Doug Scott)

Incline Press - 1 x 12
Incline Press - 2 x as many reps as possible
Supine Press - 1 x as many reps as possible
Bent-Over Row - 1 x 12 (each arm)
Lateral Raise - 1 x 12
Shrug - 1 x 15
Deadlift - 1 x 25
Crunch - 1 x 20

Performance Points:

- This workout is designed to systematically train your chest through various ranges of motion in a manner that's efficient, effective and safe. The actual workout can involve either a chest "press" (as indicated in this workout) or a chest "fly."

- Choose a weight for the first set of the incline press that allows you to perform 12 repetitions to the point of muscular fatigue.

- Do the first set of the incline press with the bench at about a 60-degree angle. For the next two sets of that exercise, lower the angle of the bench so that the second set is done at about a 45-degree angle and the third set is done at about a 30-degree angle. Finish the sequence with a set of the supine (flat bench) press. Use the same weight for all four exercises and do as many repetitions as possible (which should be about 5 - 10).

- Do the three sets of the incline press and the one set of the supine press with as little recovery as possible between each set.

- Refrain from doing this workout more than once per week since it's very demanding and requires ample recovery time.

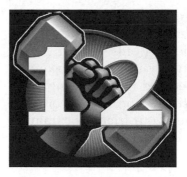

THE FINISHING TOUCH

Exercises or activities that are performed immediately after your workout are known as "finishers." Their purpose, frankly, is to "finish" you off. Finishers test your strength, conditioning and intestinal fortitude, especially at the end of your workout when your energy and stamina have been sapped from your intense efforts. Usually, finishers involve the entire body working in unison and aren't meant to target a specific muscle. But depending on the particular exercise or activity, certain muscles can take the brunt of the workload. For instance, many finishers place more demands on the posterior chain (the upper and lower back) along with the gripping muscles; others place more demands on the lower body, shoulders and stabilizer muscles.

Performing these exercises or activities places enormous demands on your musculoskeletal and cardiorespiratory systems. Indeed, you'll be huffing and puffing in no time. Plus, they make for a great adjunct to increasing your level of fitness and can add a certain aspect of enjoyment and accomplishment to your training. Although finishers are described here as a post-workout prescription, the concept can also be used for a "conditioning-only" or "strength-only" workout for added variety. By using the upcoming finishers, you can develop a specified routine using a determined weight, distance and time to provide a competitive environment, especially when your friends or training partners are involved.

STANDARD FINISHERS

Finishers can be standard exercises that may already be in your program such as the deadlift, lunge and overhead press; those that aren't standard exercises warrant further discussion. The most popular ones are the farmer's walk, dumbbell carry and stairclimbing. Here's how to do those finishers:

Farmer's Walk

Grasp a dumbbell with each hand and perform a deadlift (as described in Chapter 3). Hold the dumbbells without assistance from wrist straps or hand attachments. (This makes for excellent grip work.) In the finished position, walk a specified distance or time using a very upright posture, maintaining good form and a slow, controlled walking pace. Make sure not to lean forward or round your back as this puts undue stress on the shoulders and lower back, essentially cheating at the movement. If you choose to walk for time, you'll need to walk for that specified duration in order to obtain your goal. If you don't achieve the time, you can recover for about 10 - 20 seconds and then continue on to your destination or for the specified time. Another good means of using the farmer's walk is to do intervals of a designated distance such as 50 yards. After walking the specified distance, put down the dumbbells and take 30 seconds of recovery. Then, proceed back to the starting point until you perform the desired number of repetitions.

Dumbbell Carry

Hold the outside of the dumbbell with both hands and position your lower arms so that they're roughly parallel to the ground. Pull the dumbbell into your body and keep it in place. Use the same time/distance recommendations as the farmer's walk.

Stairclimbing

This is exactly what it sounds like. Hold the dumbbells in the same position as the farmer's walk and use the same safety guidelines but this time, carefully walk up and down stairs. Use a

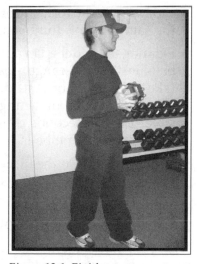

Figure 12.1: Finishers are a great way to increase the intensity of your workout and add a healthy dose of competitiveness for you and your friends.

lighter weight in this finisher than the farmer's walk. Like everything else, however, the weight should be challenging enough to provide a stimulus to the musculoskeletal and cardiorespiratory systems.

OTHER FINISHERS

Want more? Tom Kelso, the Strength Coordinator at Saint Louis University, recommends these finishers (with his colorful monikers):

- Three-Way Shoulders: Do the front raise, lateral raise and overhead press to muscular fatigue using the same pair of dumbbells.

- Fried Shoulders: Do the lateral raise, upright row and overhead press to muscular fatigue using the same pair of dumbbells.

- Grilled Shoulders: Do the front raise, lateral raise, upright row and overhead press to muscular fatigue using the same pair of dumbbells.

- Flaming Shoulders: Do a front raise and hold the dumbbells in the mid-range position for as long as possible, take 10 seconds of rest, do a lateral raise and hold the dumbbells in the mid-range position for as long as possible. Take 30 seconds of recovery and repeat using the same pair of dumbbells.

- Atomic Arms: Do the bicep curl and French curl to muscular fatigue. Repeat this sequence a total of three times with as little recovery as possible between the exercises.

SAMPLE APPLICATIONS

As previously mentioned, some standard exercises can be used to finish a workout. At the end of a hard training session, for example, you can perform a high-repetition set of the deadlift. Pick a repetition range of 50 - 100 and perform them over several minutes. Or, combine several exercises to put an entire finishing program together such as the deadlift, overhead press and farmer's walk.

Here are two examples of how you can implement finishers in your workouts:

Total-Body Workout #1 (with finishers)

Ball Squat - 1 x 20
Supine Press - 1 x 12
Bench Row - 1 x 12
Lateral Raise - 1 x 15
Shrug - 1 x 15
Bicep Curl - 1 x 12
Standing Calf Raise - 1 x 20 (each leg)
Crunch - 1 x 15
Farmer's Walk - 5 x 50 yards
Overhead Press - 1 x 50
Stairclimbing - 1 x 3 minutes

Total-Body Workout #2 (with finishers)

Overhead Press - 1 x 10 (alternating style)
Stiff-Leg Deadlift - 1 x 15
Pullover - 1 x 20
Supine Fly - 1 x 15
Bent-Over Raise - 1 x 15 (each arm)
French Curl - 1 x 12 (each arm)
Hammer Curl - 1 x 10
Seated Calf Raise - 1 x 15 (each leg)
Side Bend - 1 x 12 (each side)
Lunge - 1 x 25 (each leg)
Dumbbell Carry - 1 x 100 yards
Farmer's Walk - 1 x 100 yards

As pointed out earlier, finishers can be done to increase your level of fitness and utilized solely for conditioning purposes. For example, an obstacle course of sorts can be designed where dumbbells are placed at designated spots and you must make your way to each location to perform the next activity.

An application of this comes from Jim Bryan, the Strength Coach and Owner of Bryan Strength and Conditioning (Winter Haven, Florida). He recommends this simple but effective use of finishers:

The Medley

Farmer's Walk - 1 x 30 yards
Overhead Press - 1 x 10
Farmer's Walk - 1 x 30 yards

Performance Points:

- To do "The Medley," mark out a straight-line course of 30 yards. At one end of the course, place a pair of heavy dumbbells for the farmer's walk. At the other end of the course, place a pair of lighter dumbbells for the overhead press.

· This is a timed event and you should try to beat your time each workout. The farmer's walk is the first exercise. The time starts when you stand up with the dumbbells. Walk at a brisk pace to the far end of the course and set down the heavier dumbbells. Pick up the lighter dumbbells and perform the overhead press (while standing) for 10 repetitions. Set down the lighter dumbbells and pick up the heavier dumbbells and perform another farmer's walk to the finish line. The time ends when you cross the starting line. Repeat this sequence another 3 - 5 times, taking about 30 - 60 seconds of recovery between each series of exercises.

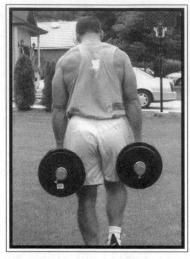

Figure 12.2: Performing exercises or activities as finishers places enormous demands on your musculoskeletal and cardiorespiratory system.

• This workout is inspired by the Strongman Competitions. Obviously, not many people will be using the weight that's normally used at strongman events. Nevertheless, the weights should be challenging but safety should be kept foremost in the mind of those doing this workout.

Here's another "all-finishers" workout from Doug Scott, the Strength and Conditioning coach at The Pingry School (Martinsville, New Jersey):

Farmer's Walk - 1 x 30 seconds
Stiff-Leg Deadlift - 1 x 15
Farmer's Walk - 1 x 30 seconds
Shrug - 1 x 20

Farmer's Walk - 1 x 30 seconds
Deadlift - 1 x 15
Farmer's Walk - 1 x 30 seconds

Performance Points:

- Use the same dumbbells for all of the exercises/activities.

THE FINISH LINE

Finishers are a great way to increase the intensity of your workout. In addition, they can add a healthy dose of competitiveness for you and your friends. And, of course, finishers can be used to improve your strength and fitness. Adding a finisher or two to your workout can truly be the finishing touch.

APPENDIX A:
Basic Anatomy – Front View

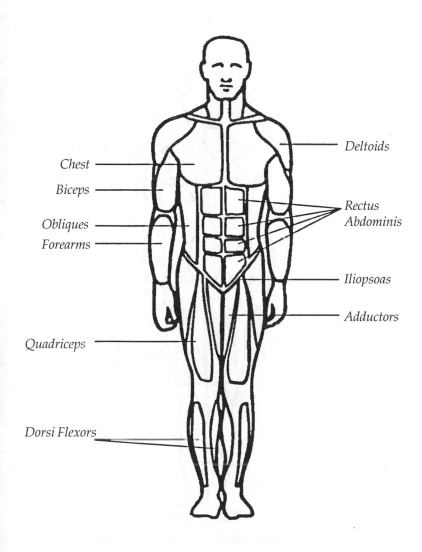

Deltoids

Chest

Biceps

Rectus
Abdominis

Obliques

Forearms

Iliopsoas

Adductors

Quadriceps

Dorsi Flexors

APPENDIX B:
Basic Anatomy – Back View

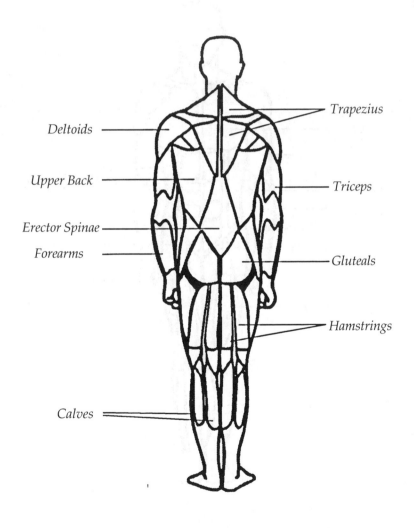

Deltoids

Upper Back

Erector Spinae

Forearms

Trapezius

Triceps

Gluteals

Hamstrings

Calves

THE CONTRIBUTORS

Almost of the workouts that appear throughout the book were provided courtesy of the following individuals. The authors appreciate their valuable contributions not only to this book but also to the strength and fitness profession.

Steve Baldwin, Strength Coach and Owner
Just Strength Training
Nashville, Tennessee

Drew Baye
Baye Fitness
Altamonte Springs, Florida
www.baye.com

Randy Berning, Owner
Brickwise Training Center
Cincinnati, Ohio

Michael Bradley, Strength and Conditioning Coach (Basketball)
Florida State University
Tallahassee, Florida

Jim Bryan, Strength Coach and Owner
Bryan Strength and Conditioning
Winter Haven, Florida
www.hometown.aol.com/macthai/myhomepagebusiness.html

Luke Carlson, Owner
Discover Strength, Inc.
Minneapolis, Minnesota

Brian Conatser, Strength and Conditioning Coach
Sycamore High School
Cincinnati, Ohio

Michael De Joseph, P.E. Teacher and Football Coach
Babylon High School
Babylon, New York

Jeff Friday, Strength and Conditioning Coach
Baltimore Ravens
Owings Mils, Maryland

Jason Hadeed, President
Elite Athlete Training Systems, Inc.
Rockville, Maryland
www.EliteAthleteTraining.com
www.StrengthConference.com

Chip Harrison, Strength and Conditioning Coach
The Pennsylvania State University
University Park, Pennsylvania

Aaron Hillman, Strength and Conditioning Coach
Bowling Green State University
Bowling Green, Ohio

Gregg Humphreys, Head Coach of Judo and Sambo
Miletich Fighting Systems
Davenport, Iowa

Sunir Jossan, Chief Fitness Branch
National CounterTerrorism Center
Washington, DC
www.thepersonaledge.net

Tom Kelso, Coordinator of Strength and Conditioning
Saint Louis University
Saint Louis, Missouri
www.tomkelso.com

Dr. Paul Kennedy, Strength and Fitness Consultant
Phoenix, Arizona
www.befitstayfit.com

Sam Knopik, Head Football Coach
Pembroke Hill School
Kansas City, Missouri
www.StrongerAthlete.com

Aaron R. Komarek, Vice President
Director of Athletics and Sports Performance
Sports + Field at Seven Oaks
Wesley Chapel, Florida

Kristopher R. Kotch, Exercise Specialist
The Heart Hospital
Geisinger Wyoming Valley
Wilkes-Barre, Pennsylvania

Mike Lawrence, Head Strength Coach
Missouri Southern State University
Joplin, Missouri

Dr. Ken Leistner, Strength Coach
Valley Stream, New York

Ken Mannie, Strength and Conditioning Coach
Michigan State University
East Lansing, Michigan

John Mikula, Sports Performance Strength and Conditioning
Memphis, Tennessee

Willis Paine, Fitness Director
Kokopelli Fitness Center
Princeton, New Jersey

Adam Rankin, Strength and Conditioning Coach
Archbishop Elder High School
Cincinnati, Ohio

Jeff Roudebush, Head Track Coach and Assistant Football Coach
Pembroke Hill School
Kansas City, Missouri
www.StrongerAthlete.com

Doug Scott, Strength Coach
The Pingry School
Martinsville, New Jersey

Mike Shibinski, Strength and Conditioning Coach
Princeton High School
Cincinnati, Ohio

Rob Spector, Author of the HIT FAQ
Atlanta, Georgia
www.cyberpump.com

Scott Swanson, Strength Coach
U. S. Military Academy
West Point, New York

ABOUT THE AUTHORS

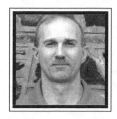 **MATT BRZYCKI**, B.S., is the Coordinator of Recreational Fitness and Wellness Programs at Princeton University in Princeton, New Jersey. He has more than 22 years of experience at the collegiate level as a coach, instructor and administrator. His current responsibilities at Princeton University include managing the Stephens Fitness Center and teaching a variety of fitness classes such as Adult Fitness, Introduction to Free Weights, Introductory Strength Training and Women-n-Weights.

Matt served in the United States Marine Corps from 1975-79 which included a 12-month tour of duty as a Drill Instructor. He earned his Bachelor of Science degree in Health and Physical Education from Penn State in 1983.

He has been a featured speaker at local, regional, state and national conferences, clinics and sports camps throughout the United States and Canada. This includes presentations at the U. S. Secret Service Academy; the Princeton University Strength & Speed Camp; the National Strength & Science Seminar; the American College of Sports Medicine's Health & Fitness Summit & Exposition; the Tampa Bay Buccaneer Strength and Conditioning Seminar; and the Toronto Football Clinic. He developed a correspondence course for Desert Southwest Fitness (Tucson, Arizona) that was used by strength and fitness professionals to update their certifications and co-developed a SWAT (Special Weapons and Tactics) Fitness Specialist Certification Program for law-enforcement and military personnel. Matt has written more than 285 articles/columns on strength and fitness that have been featured in 41 different publications. In addition, he has authored, co-authored or edited 14 books.

Matt developed the Strength Training Theory and Applications class and taught the course to Exercise Science and Sport Studies majors at Rutgers University as a member of the Faculty of Arts and Sciences from 1990-2000. He also developed the Weight Training class and taught the course to Health and Physical Education majors and other students at The College of New Jersey as a member of the Health and Physical Education Faculty from 1996-1999.

Matt was appointed by the governor to serve on the New Jersey Council on Physical Fitness and Sports as well as the New Jersey Obesity Prevention Task Force. He was elected to serve on the Alumni Society Board of Directors for the College of Health & Human Development (Penn State) and is the chair of its Awards Committee. Matt and his wife, Alicia, reside in Lawrenceville, New Jersey, with their son, Ryan.

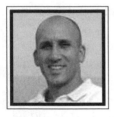 **FRED FORNICOLA**, B.A., is the President and exclusive personal trainer of Premiere Personal Fitness *(www.premierepersonalfitness.com)* in Asbury Park, New Jersey. In addition, he serves as a fitness equipment consultant for schools and corporations for Fitness Lifestyles, Inc. as well as the fitness professional who oversees Newberry Fitness (also of Asbury Park).

Fred has been involved in the field of strength and fitness for nearly 30 years. He has authored more than 75 articles on strength and fitness while maintaining several regular columns on nutrition and training for numerous Internet websites. Also, he's the Editor-in-Chief of the *High Performance Training* newsletter and has been published in periodicals such as *Master Trainer* and *Hardgainer*. In addition, he's a contributing author of the book *Get Fit New Jersey!* Fred serves as a resource member of the New Jersey Council on Physical Fitness and Sports.

He received his Bachelor of Arts degree in Business from Stockton College in 1983. Fred and his wife, Lori, reside in Oakhurst, New Jersey, with their daughter, Alexa.